AF483527

Pharmaceutics
A Practical Manual
Third Edition

Pharmaceutics
A Practical Manual
Third Edition

Sindhu Abraham

Assistant Professor,
Department of Pharmaceutics,
M.S Ramaiah College of Pharmacy,
Bangalore.

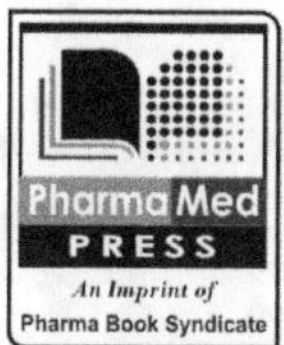

PharmaMed Press
An imprint of Pharma Book Syndicate
A unit of BSP Books Pvt., Ltd.
4-4-309/316, Giriraj Lane,
Sultan Bazar, Hyderabad - 500 095.

Published by

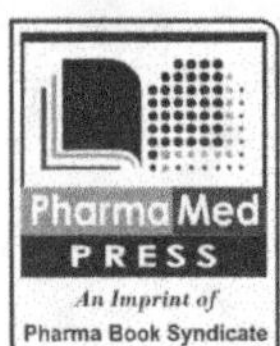

PharmaMed Press

An imprint of Pharma Book Syndicate

A unit of BSP Books Pvt. Ltd.

4-4-309/316, Giriraj Lane, Sultan Bazar, Hyderabad - 500 095.

Phone: 040-23445688, 23445600; Fax: 91+40-23445611

E-mail: info@pharmamedpress.com

www.pharmamedpress.com/pharmamedpress.net

ISBN: 978-93-88305-08-2

Preface to Third Edition

Pharmaceutics is a branch of pharmacy concerned with the art and science of dosage form design. The word Pharmaceutics comprises varied subject areas that are associated with the steps involved in formulation development.

There are a number of practical manuals in Pharmaceutics which caters to the needs of B.Pharm and D.Pharm students. This comprehensive manual is a sincere effort to provide practical knowledge in Pharmaceutics for Pharm.D, B.Pharm and D. Pharm students and has been prepared in accordance with the syllabus prescribed by the PCI.

The manual encompasses chapters covering all conventional dosage forms such as syrups, elixirs, solutions, liniments, suspensions, emulsions, powders, suppositories etc. Experiments on incompatibilities have also been included.

Special emphasis has been laid on:

(a) Concepts and principles of each experiment.

(b) Synonym / Latin terms for selected preparations.

(c) Marketed formulations available for certain preparations

(d) Appendices as ready reckoner.

(e) Question bank containing frequently asked questions.

Further suggestions and criticism from teachers and students will be highly appreciated.

- Author

Acknowledgements

I express my deep sense of gratitude to Dr. V. Madhavan, Principal, M. S Ramaiah College of Pharmacy, Bangalore for his constant support and encouragement.

My sincere thanks to Dr. S. Bharath, Professor and HOD, Dr. B. V Basavaraj, Associate Professor, Dr. R. Deveswaran, Associate Professor, Mrs. Sharon Furtado, Assistant Professor and Mrs. Shwetha, Assistant Professor, Department of Pharmaceutics, M. S Ramaiah College of Pharmacy, for their unceasing support, assistance and encouragement in bringing out the revised edition of this book. It is their inspiration that has helped me go ahead with the preparation of this work.

I also thank M/s Pharma Book Syndicate for publishing this book and in particular Mr. Anil Shah and Mr. Naresh Davergave for their enthusiasm and support in printing this book.

- Author

Contents

Format for Record Writing

The details to be written in the left hand side of the record include:
1. Calculations
2. Label

The details to be written in the right hand side of the record include:
1. Name of the Preparation
2. Aim
3. Synonym (if any)
4. Formula
5. Principle
6. Procedure
7. Category
8. Dose
9. Directions
10. Auxiliary label
11. Storage

The format for the label will be as follows

Quantity of the Preparation : in ml /g/ numbers
NAME OF THE PREPARATION (IP/BP/BPC/NF)
SYNONYM: Another name for the preparation
DRUG Content: Name and quantity of the active ingredient(s)
CATEGORY: Use of the preparation
DOSAGE: (If any or write "As directed by the Physician")
DIRECTIONS: On how to use the preparation
AUXILIARY LABEL: Includes precautions to be taken while administering the preparation. To be written in red, bold letters
Storage: Condition at which the preparation should be stored
Mfg. Date :   **Exp. Date :** **Batch no:**   **Mfg. Lic. No:** **Mfd. By:** **M.R.P**

Syrups

Syrups are sweet, viscous, concentrated solutions of sucrose or other sugars in water or any other suitable aqueous vehicle. The pharmacopoeial syrups have a high concentration of sucrose (66.7%w/w according to IP and 85%w/v according to USP) which is necessary for stability. Stronger solutions tend to crystallize and more dilute solutions support microbial growth.

The aqueous sugar medium of dilute sucrose solutions is an efficient nutrient medium for the growth of microorganisms, particularly yeasts and moulds whereas, concentrated sugar solutions are quite resistant to microbial growth because of their high osmotic pressure.

Simple syrup requires no additional preservative if it is to be used soon. Preservatives are added if the syrup is to be stored. When properly prepared and maintained, the syrup is inherently stable and resistant to the growth of microorganisms. As formulated, the official syrup is both stable and resistant to microbial growth & crystallization. However commercial syrups must employ preservatives to prevent microbial growth and to ensure their stability during their period of use and storage.

Syrups should be stored at constant temperature, since fluctuations encourage crystallization and in well closed containers to prevent entry of moisture. Moisture can dilute the surface layer, allow microorganisms to multiply and fermentation occurs.

There are two types of syrups:

1. ***Non medicated or Flavoured syrups:*** These syrups contain flavouring agents but not medicinal substances. They are intended to serve as pleasant tasting vehicles for medicated syrups.

   E.g. Orange syrup, Lemon syrup, Cocoa syrup, Raspberry syrup, Cherry syrup.

2. ***Medicated syrups:*** These preparations contain medicinal substance/s along with the other additives.

   E.g. Ephedrine hydrochloride syrup, Paracetamol syrup.

Syrups provide a pleasant means of administering a liquid preparation containing a disagreeable tasting drug. They are particularly effective in the administration of drugs to children.

Syrups may contain a small concentration of alcohol as a preservative or as a solvent to incorporate flavouring agents.

Preparation of Syrups

Syrups may be prepared by one of the following methods, depending on the physical and chemical character of the ingredients:

1. ***Solution with the aid of heat:*** This method is used when the ingredients of the syrup are not volatile in nature and are heat stable. The sugar is added to the purified water and heated until is completely dissolved. Other heat stable ingredients are then mixed with the hot syrup and made upto volume. The use of heat facilitates faster solution of sugar and other ingredients.

   The disadvantage of this method is that heating may lead to the inversion of sucrose. The sweetness of the syrup will be altered, because invert sugar is sweeter than sucrose. The decomposed syrup attains a dark coloration due to caramellization and is more susceptible to fermentation and microbial growth.

2. ***Solution by agitation without the aid of heat:*** this method is used when the ingredients are heat sensitive and to prevent heat induced inversion of sucrose.

   All the ingredients are dissolved in purified water by continuous agitation.

3. ***Addition of sucrose to a medicated or flavoured liquid:*** In this method, sucrose is added to the medicated liquid, which may be a tincture or an extract.

4. ***Percolation:*** In the percolation method, the medicinal agent may be percolated to form an extract, to which sucrose or syrup is added.

   E.g. Ipecac syrup is prepared by adding glycerin and syrup to an extractive of powdered ipecac obtained by percolation.

EXPERIMENT 1

Simple Syrup IP

Aim

To prepare and submit 20 g of Simple syrup.

Formula

Sl. No	Ingredients	Official formula	Working formula
1	Sucrose	667g	
2	Purified water (q.s)	1000g	

Principle

Syrups are sweet, viscous, concentrated solutions of sucrose or other sugars in water or any other suitable aqueous vehicle. The pharmacopoeial syrups have a high concentration of sucrose (66.7 % W/W according to IP or approx 85%W/V according to U.S.P), which is necessary for stability.

Stronger solutions tend to crystallize and dilute solutions can support microbial growth. Therefore at 66.7%W/W, simple syrup acts as a self-preservative. The self-preservative activity of syrup is attributed to the high osmotic pressure.

Syrups should be stored at a constant temperature to prevent crystallization and in well-closed containers to prevent entry of moisture.

Moisture can dilute the surface layer and may allow microorganisms to multiply and fermentation may occur.

Procedure

1. A 100ml empty beaker was weighed and the weight was noted.

2. Half the quantity of purified water was placed in to the beaker. Calculated quantity of sucrose was weighed and added to the water.

3. Sucrose was dissolved by heating with occasional stirring.

4. After cooling, purified water was added to make up the required weight.

Category

Pharmaceutical aid (Vehicle) and sweetening agent.

Storage

Store in a cool and dry place.

EXPERIMENT 2

Orange Syrup BPC

Aim

To prepare and submit 20 ml of Orange Syrup.

Synonym

Syrup of orange peel / Syrupus Aurantii.

Formula

Sl. No	Ingredients	Official formula	Working formula
1	Tincture of orange	60ml	
2	Simple syrup (q.s)	1000ml	

Principle

Tincture of orange is an alcoholic extract of fresh bitter orange peels and is prepared by maceration process. Fresh peel is used for this preparation because it is stable and contains a higher proportion of volatile oil than the dried peels. Drying dissipates part of the oil and fresh peels are more aromatic. Alcohol (90%) is used as the menstruum for the maceration process.

This preparation contains flavouring oils which are volatile in nature and should therefore be stored in tightly closed containers in a cool place.

Procedure

1. The measured quantity of orange tincture was mixed with 3/4th the quantity of simple syrup.

2. The volume was then made up with the remaining syrup.

Category

Pleasant acidic vehicle, carminative, flavoring and sweetening agent.

Dose

2 - 4 ml

Storage

Store in a cool and dry place.

EXPERIMENT 3

Orange Syrup NF

Aim

To prepare and submit 20 ml of Orange Syrup.

Formula

Sl. No	Ingredients	Official formula	Working formula
1	Sweet orange peel tincture	50ml	
2	Sucrose	820g	
3	Talc	15g	
4	Anhydrous citric acid	5g	
5	Purified water (q.s)	1000ml	

Principle

Orange syrup is prepared by dissolving sucrose in an aqueous solution of orange oil and citric acid. Sweet orange peel tincture NF is used as the source of the oil. The syrup is employed as a flavoured vehicle.

Procedure

1. The talc was triturated with the tincture and citric acid.
2. 400ml of purified water was gradually added. The mixture was filtered, returning the first portions of the filtrate until it becomes clear. Enough purified water was added to make the filtrate measure 450ml.

3. The sucrose was dissolved in the filtrate by agitation without heating.
4. Sufficient quantity of water was then added to make the product measure 1000ml.

Category

Pleasant acidic vehicle, carminative, flavoring and sweetening agent.

Dose

4 – 5 ml to be taken thrice a day.

Storage

Store in a cool and dry place.

EXPERIMENT 4

Ephedrine Hydrochloride Syrup NF

Aim

To prepare and submit 20 ml of Ephedrine Hydrochloride syrup.

Formula

Sl.No	Ingredients	Official formula	Working formula
1	Ephedrine Hydrochloride	4 g	
2	Sucrose	800 g	
3	Ethyl alcohol	25 ml	
4	Amaranth Solution	4 ml	
5	Citric acid	1 g	
6	Caramel	0.4 g	
7	Lemon oil	0.25ml	
8	Orange oil	0.25ml	
9	Benzaldehyde	0.016ml	
10	Purified water (q.s)	1000ml	

Principle

Ephedrine hydrochloride is an alkaloidal salt used as a bronchodilator in asthma and also in the treatment of allergic conditions like hay fever. Sucrose is used to increase the viscosity and sweetness of the preparation. Citric acid, an organic acid is used as a buffer to maintain the final pH of the preparation. Amaranth solution is the coloring agent. Caramel is burnt sugar and is used as coloring and sweetening agent. Lemon oil and orange oil are flavoring agents. Benzaldehyde is a preservative. Ethyl alcohol is a co-solvent and is used to dissolve lemon oil and orange oil. It also acts as a preservative.

Procedure

1. The weighed quantity of Sucrose was dissolved in a minimum quantity of hot water.

2. To the above solution Benzaldehyde, Ephedrine Hydrochloride, citric acid and caramel were added slowly with constant stirring.

3. Orange oil and Lemon oil was dissolved in alcohol and added to the above solution. Amaranth solution was also added.

4. The solution was then made up to the volume with purified water.

Category

Bronchodilator.

Dose

5-10ml (each 5ml will contain 20mg of Ephedrine hydrochloride).

Storage

Store in a well closed container in a cool and dry place.

EXPERIMENT 5

Vasaka Syrup IP

Aim

To prepare and submit 20 ml of Vasaka Syrup.

Formula

Sl.No	Ingredients	Official formula	Working formula
1	Vasaka liquid extract	500ml	
2	Glycerin	100ml	
3	Syrup (q.s)	1000ml	

Principle

Vasaka consists of the dried as well as fresh leaves of the plant *Adhatoda vasica*. Vasaka is used as an expectorant and bronchodilator.

Procedure

The Vasaka liquid extract was mixed with glycerin and made upto volume with syrup.

Category

Expectorant and Bronchodilator.

Dose

2-4 ml

Storage

Store in a cool and dry place.

Marketed Formulations

VASAKA SYRUP (Kudos Laboratories)

VASAKA SYRUP (Unijules Life sciences Ltd.)

EXPERIMENT 6

Ferrous Phosphate Syrup IP

Aim

To prepare and submit 20 ml of Ferrous Phosphate Syrup.

Synonym

Parrish's food, Parrish's syrup, Chemical food, Syrupus ferri Phosphatis.

(According to BPC 1968 this preparation is called Compound Ferrous Phosphate syrup and the synonyms are *Parrish's food, Parrish's syrup, Chemical food, Syrupus ferri Phosphatis Compositus*)

Formula

Sl. No	Ingredients	Official formula	Working formula
1	Sucrose	700g	
2	Calcium carbonate	13.6g	
3	Iron filings	4.3g	
4	Cochineal	3.5g	
5	Potassium bicarbonate	1g	
6	Sodium phosphate	1g	
7	Orange flower water of commerce (undiluted)	50ml	
8	Phosphoric acid	48 ml	
9	Purified water (q.s)	1000ml	

Principle

An insufficient supply of iron in the diet may lead to a condition called anemia. In such conditions, ferrous phosphate syrup is prescribed as an iron supplement. This preparation contains iron along with electrolytes like Ca^{2+}, K^+ and Na^+. These electrolytes overcome the deficiencies which are most common in anaemic condition.

Electrolytes can also be supplied in their phosphate form and are obtained by reaction between phosphoric acid, calcium carbonate, potassium bicarbonate and sodium phosphate.

This syrup is made by chemical interaction.

1. ***First stage:*** is the preparation of a solution of ferrous acid phosphate.

   Iron filings, phosphoric acid and water are heated in a flask on a water bath until the iron dissolves.

   $$Fe + 2\,H_3PO_4 \longrightarrow Fe[H_2PO_4]_2 + \uparrow H_2$$
   Ferrous acid phosphate

   Heating over a water bath is specified to minimize volatilization of water – if the reaction mixture becomes dry or even approaches dryness. A solid block is formed which does not dissolve when water is added. Oxidation during heating cannot occur as long as hydrogen (H_2) is being evolved.

2. ***Second stage:*** is the preparation of a solution containing phosphoric acid, calcium carbonate, potassium bicarbonate, sodium phosphate and purified water, which is mixed in a capacious vessel.

   $$CaCO_3 + 2\,H_3PO_4 \longrightarrow Ca[H_2PO_4]_2 + CO_2 \uparrow + H_2O$$
   Calcium Phosphate

   $$KHCO_3 + H_3PO_4 \longrightarrow KH_2PO_4 + CO_2 \uparrow + H_2O$$
   Potassium Phosphate

   $$Na_2HPO_4 + H_3PO_4 \longrightarrow 2Na\,H_2PO_4$$
   Sodium Phosphate

   At this stage there is insufficient phosphoric acid to complete the reaction. Hence excess of phosphoric acid is added to complete the reactions. Evolution of CO_2 is considerable; hence a capacious vessel is necessary.

The iron and calcium solutions are then mixed and filtered. The mixture is filtered to remove iron carbide and carbon derived from the iron solution.

3. ***Third stage:*** is the preparation of a colored syrup containing cochineal, sucrose and distilled water. The cochineal is extracted by decoction process. The cochineal is used whole to facilitate straining. Reboiling after addition of the sugar ensures that the finished product will not ferment. An uncolored product in this syrup would be pale green when freshly prepared but would soon become reddish brown due to oxidation. The cochineal conceals this change.

The orange flower water flavors the preparation.

Procedure

1. Phosphoric acid was diluted with water. This was divided into two portions.

2. To one portion of diluted phosphoric acid, iron filings were added. The contents were heated on a water bath until the iron is completely dissolved.

3. Calcium carbonate, potassium bicarbonate and sodium phosphate were dissolved in the second portion of diluted phosphoric acid in a beaker by continuous stirring. CO_2 was allowed to evolve.

4. The iron phosphate solution was mixed with the above solution.

5. The resulting solution was filtered to remove impurities like iron carbide and carbon derived from the iron solution.

6. Cochineal was boiled in water for 15 min. Sucrose was added and the heating continued until sucrose dissolved completely. The hot syrup was cooled, strained and washed with water to produce a specified volume.

7. Into this syrup, the solution containing iron phosphate, calcium carbonate, potassium bicarbonate and sodium phosphate were added and mixed well.

8. Orange flower water was then added and the solution was made upto the volume with purified water. The solution was then allowed to stand for 48 hours and filtered if necessary.

Category

Calcium and iron tonic (Haematinic).

Dose

2 - 8 ml or (2.5 – 10 ml).

Storage

Store in a cool and dark place.

Elixirs

Elixirs are clear, flavoured, sweetened hydroalcoholic liquid oral preparations of potent or nauseous drugs. They are pleasantly flavoured and attractively coloured.

There are two types of elixirs:

1. ***Non Medicated elixirs:*** These elixirs contain flavouring agents but not medicinal substances. They are employed as vehicles for other liquid preparations.

> E.g., Compound Benzaldehyde elixir

2. ***Medicated elixirs:*** are used for the therapeutic effect of the medicinal agents they contain.

> E.g., Phenobarbital elixir, Theophylline elixir.

Medicated elixirs contain potent and nauseous drugs like antibiotic, antihistaminics, antitussives and sedatives. The bitter and nauseous taste of these drugs is masked by the presence of flavouring and sweetening agents in hydroalcoholic medium.

Compared to syrups, elixirs are usually less sweet and less viscous because they contain a lower proportion of sugar and consequently are less effective than syrups in masking the taste of medicinal substances. Due to the presence of alcohol in elixirs, the solubility of drug and other volatile ingredients is enhanced.

The proportion of alcohol in elixirs varies according to the individual ingredients. In addition to alcohol and water, other solvents like glycerin and propylene glycol are also employed as co-solvents. Elixirs may be sweetened with sucrose, sucrose syrup, sorbitol, glycerin and / or artificial sweeteners.

Preparations having a high alcoholic content usually use an artificial sweetener such as saccharin, which is required only in small amounts than sucrose which is slightly soluble in alcohol and requires greater quantities.

Formulation

1. Vehicles – Purified water, glycerin
2. Sweetening agents- Sucrose, Saccharin
3. Colouring agents – Tartrazine, Amaranth
4. Flavoring agents – Peppermint spirit, Raspberry juice, Anise water
5. Preservatives- chloroform spirit

Storage

Because of their usual content of alcohol and volatile oils, elixirs should be stored in tight, light resistant containers and protected from excessive heat.

Differences between syrups & elixirs

Sl.No	Syrups	Elixirs
1.	Syrups are sweet, viscous, concentrated solutions of sucrose or other sugars in water or any other suitable aqueous vehicle	Elixirs are clear, flavoured, sweetened hydroalcoholic solution liquid oral preparations of potent or nauseous drugs.
2.	Syrups are more sweet in nature	Sweetness is relatively less
3.	Syrups have high viscosity	Elixirs have less viscosity
4.	Alcohol is not added or the content will be very less.	Alcohol content varies from 4 – 40%
5.	Syrups can be used as sweetening agents for other formulations	Elixirs are not used as sweetening agents.

Marketed Formulations

BENADRYL (Johnson & Johnson)

NOVAKUF (Lupin)

BROMHEXINE Elixir (IPCA)

FESOVIT (GSK)

RUBRAPLEX (Piramal Health care)

Piperazine Citrate Elixir BPC

Aim

To prepare and submit 20 ml of Piperazine citrate elixir.

Synonym

Elixir Piperazinae Citratis.

Formula

Sl.No	Ingredients	Official formula	Working formula
1	Piperazine citrate	187.5 g	
2	Syrup	500 ml	
3	Glycerin	100 ml	
4	Green S and Tartrazine solution	15 ml	
5	Peppermint spirit	5 ml	
6	Purified Water (q.s)	1000 ml	

Principle

Elixirs are clear, flavoured, sweetened hydroalcoholic liquid oral preparations of potent or nauseous drugs.

They are pleasantly flavoured and attractively coloured.

Piperazine Citrate is an anthelmintic. Syrup is used as the sweetener to mask the bitter taste of piperazine citrate and also to increase the viscosity of the preparation. Glycerin is used to increase the viscosity of the preparation. Green S and Tartrazine solution is the coloring agent. Peppermint spirit is the flavoring agent.

Procedure

1. Piperazine citrate was dissolved in a small portion of purified water.
2. Green S and tartrazine solution, glycerin, syrup and peppermint spirit are then added to the above solution with continuous stirring.
3. Sufficient purified water was then added to produce the required volume.

Category

Anthelmintic.

Dose

Adult: For threadworm infestations: 15ml daily

As an ascaricide: 30ml as a single dose

Child: For threadworm infestations: 9months – 2 yrs: 2.5ml daily

2 - 3 yrs: 5 ml daily

4 – 6 yrs: 7.5 ml daily

7 – 12 yrs: 10ml daily

Storage

Store in a cool place away from light.

EXPERIMENT 8

Paediatric Paracetamol Elixir BPC

Aim

To prepare and submit 20 ml of Paediatric Paracetamol elixir.

Synonym

Elixir Paracetamolis pro Infantibus.

Formula

Sl.No	Ingredients	Official formula	Working formula
1	Paracetamol	24 g	
2	Invert syrup	275 ml	
3	Alcohol (95%)	100 ml	
4	Propylene glycol	100 ml	
5	Concentrated Raspberry Juice	25 ml	
6	Chloroform Spirit	20 ml	
7	Amaranth Solution	2 ml	
8	Glycerin (q.s)	1000 ml	

Principle

This is a preparation containing 2.4%w/v of Paracetamol in a suitable flavoured vehicle. Paracetamol acts as an analgesic and anti-pyretic with mild anti- inflammatory activity. Since Paracetamol is sparingly soluble in water, alcohol and propylene glycol are used to increase its solubility.

Invert syrup contains a mixture of glucose & fructose and may be prepared by hydrolyzing sucrose with a mineral acid such as hydrochloric acid and neutralizing the solution with Calcium carbonate or Sodium carbonate. Invert syrup when mixed in suitable proportions with syrup, prevents the deposition of crystals of sucrose under most conditions of storage. It is also used as the sweetening agent to mask the bitter taste of the drug.

Chloroform spirit is the preservative. Raspberry juice is the flavoring agent. Amaranth solution is the coloring agent. Glycerin is the vehicle and also increases the viscosity of the preparation.

Procedure

1. Paracetamol was dissolved in a mixture of alcohol, propylene glycol and chloroform spirit with stirring.
2. Conc. Raspberry juice dissolved in invert syrup and amaranth solution were added to the above solution and mixed well.
3. Sufficient glycerin was added to produce the required volume.

Category

Analgesic and Anti-pyretic.

Dose

Upto 1yr: 5ml (each 5ml of the preparation will contain 120mg of Paracetamol).

1 to 5 yrs: 10ml (each 10ml of the preparation will contain 240mg of Paracetamol).

Auxiliary label

Do not dilute with water.

Storage

Protect from light.

EXPERIMENT 9

Cascara Elixir BP

Aim

To prepare and submit 20 ml of Cascara Elixir.

Synonym

Cascara Sagrada elixir.

Formula

Sl.No	Ingredients	Official formula	Working formula
1	Cascara (coarse powder)	1000g	
2	Liquorice (coarse powder)	125g	
3	Light magnesium oxide	50g	
4	Saccharin sodium	1g	
5	Glycerin	300 ml	
6	Alcohol (90%)	12.5 ml	
7	Coriander oil	0.15ml	
8	Anise oil	0.2 ml	
9	Purified water (q.s)	1000 ml	

Principle

Cascara coarse powder is obtained from the bark of *Cascara Sagrada*. It is a hard drug an its constituents are readily water soluble. Hence water is used as a menstruum for percolation and coarse powder of the crude drug is used.

The ingredients of cascara have a nauseating odour and persistently bitter in taste. Hence sweetening agents are added to mask the bitter taste. Eg. Saccharin sodium & glycyrrhizin.

Glycyrrhizin is present in liquorice root and is water soluble. Hence unpeeled pieces of root of liquorice are used.

Light magnesium oxide converts the bitter substance lactone present in *Cascara Sagrada* into a less bitter magnesium salt.

Corainder and anise oils are used as flavouring agents to mask the odour of the drug. These oils are soluble in alcohol. In this preparation, glycerin is used to increase viscosity and as a sweetening agent.

Purified water is used as the menstruum. Percolation is conducted at or near 100^0C, so the proteins in liquorice gets precipitated which remain in the tissue. As a result, the percolate obtained is practically free from protein.

Procedure

1. Weighed quantities of Cascara, Liquorice and light magnesium oxide were mixed.
2. 1250 ml of boiling purified water was added to the above blend and stirred thoroughly.
3. The mixture was macerated for 24 hours in a well covered vessel. During this period, the tissue swells and the magnesium oxide reacts with lactone.
4. The moistened powder mixture was packed tightly in a percolator. Boiling purified water was added to the percolator for extracting the active principles. Percolation was continued until the drug was exhausted, which is indicated by an almost colourless percolate. This can be confirmed by the following test:

Test	Observation	Inference	Instruction
A few drops of percolate + a few drops of 5 % potassium hydroxide solution	Red colour appears	Active principles present	Continue percolation
	Absence of red colour	Active principles absent	Stop percolation

1. The percolate was then evaporated to about 650 ml on a water bath. The saccharin sodium was dissolved in 12 ml purified water and the coriander and anise oils are dissolved in 90% alcohol.
2. Both solutions were mixed with glycerin and the concentrated percolate was added.
3. Sufficient purified water was added to produce 1000ml and shaken thoroughly.
4. The elixir was allowed to stand for not less than 12 hours and filtered.

Category

Purgative.

Dose

2 - 4 ml.

Storage

Store in a cool and dry place.

Linctuses

Linctuses are viscous, liquid preparations used for the treatment or relief of cough. The vehicle is always syrup and this by soothing the sore mucous membranes of the throat, has a beneficial effect. To obtain prolonged action; linctuses should be taken undiluted, sipped and swallowed slowly.

Linctuses should be stored at a constant temperature to prevent crystallization and in well-closed containers to prevent entry of moisture. Moisture can dilute the surface layer and may allow microorganisms to multiply and fermentation may occur.

The usual dose is 5ml and part doses must be diluted to this volume. The diluent is syrup, except for Diabetic codeine linctus for which chloroform water is used.

Formulation

1. Vehicles – Simple syrup, chloroform water (for Diabetic codeine linctus).
2. Colouring agents – Tartrazine, Amaranth.
3. Flavoring agents – Anise water, Peppermint water, Lemon syrup.
4. Preservatives – Chloroform Spirit.

Auxiliary Label

TO BE SIPPED AND SWALLOWED SLOWLY WITHOUT DILUTION WITH WATER.

Marketed Formulations

MIT'S LINCTUS CODEINE (Astra Zeneca)

MIT'S LINCTUS-DX (Astra Zeneca)

SINAREST LINCTUS (Centaur)

DIAKOF (Himalaya)

CONTUS PAED LINCTUS (Stedman)

EXPERIMENT 10

Simple Linctus BPC

Aim

To prepare and submit 20 ml of Simple Linctus.

Synonym

Linctus Simplex.

Formula

Sl.No	Ingredients	Official formula	Working formula
1	Citric acid	25 g	
2	Chloroform spirit	60 ml	
3	Amaranth solution	15 ml	
4	Concentrated Anise water	10 ml	
5	Simple syrup (q.s)	1000ml	

Principle

Linctuses are sweetened, viscous liquid preparations usually prescribed for the relief of cough. They contain a high concentration of sucrose, which has a demulcent action on the mucous membranes of the throat. Linctuses should be sipped and swallowed slowly and should not be diluted before use in order to obtain contact between the drug and mucous membrane of the throat for a longer period of time.

In the following preparation, Citric acid is an expectorant, demulcent and flavoring agent. Concentrated Anise water is an expectorant, carminative and flavoring agent. Chloroform spirit is the preservative. Amaranth solution is the colouring agent. Simple syrup is used as the vehicle and also to increase the viscosity of the preparation.

Procedure

1. Citric acid was dissolved in concentrated anise water.
2. Amaranth solution and Chloroform spirit was added to the above solution.
3. Syrup was then added to make up the required volume.

Category

Demulcent (to relieve sore throat).

Dose

5 ml

Direction

To be sipped and swallowed slowly.

Do not dilute with water.

Storage

Store in a cool and dry place.

EXPERIMENT 11

Paediatric Simple Linctus BPC

Aim

To prepare and submit 20 ml of Paediatric Simple Linctus.

Synonym

Linctus Simplex pro Infantibus.

Formula

Sl.No	Ingredients	Official formula	Working formula
1	Simple Linctus	250 ml	
2	Syrup (q.s)	1000ml	

Principle

Paediatric simple linctus is used in children as a demulcent and expectorant for the treatment of cough. Children require lower doses than adults. Therefore simple linctus is diluted with simple syrup to prepare paediatric simple linctus.

Procedure

Simple linctus and syrup were mixed to form paediatric simple linctus.

Category

Demulcent (to relieve sore throat).

Dose

5 - 10 ml

Direction

To be sipped and swallowed slowly.
 Do not dilute with water.

Storage

Store in a cool and dry place.

Codeine Linctus BPC

Aim

To prepare and submit 20 ml of Codeine Linctus.

Formula

Sl. No	Ingredients	Official formula	Working formula
1	Codeine Phosphate	3 g	
2	Compound Tartrazine solution	10 ml	
3	Benzoic acid solution	20 ml	
4	Chloroform spirit	20 ml	
5	Purified water	20 ml	
6	Lemon syrup	200 ml	
7	Syrup (q.s)	1000 ml	

Principle

Linctuses are sweetened, viscous liquid preparations usually prescribed for the relief of cough. They contain a high concentration of sucrose, which has a demulcent action on the mucous membranes of the throat. Linctuses should be sipped and swallowed slowly and should not be diluted before use in order to obtain contact between the drug and mucous membrane of the throat for a longer period of time.

In the following preparation, Codeine Phosphate is an anti-tussive. Lemon syrup is the flavoring agent. Benzoic acid solution and Chloroform spirit are the preservatives Compound tartrazine solution is the colouring agent. Syrup is used as the vehicle and also to increase the viscosity of the preparation.

Procedure

1. Codeine Phosphate was dissolved in water.

2. 500 ml of the syrup was added to it and mixed well.

3. Compound tartrazine solution, benzoic acid solution, chloroform spirit and lemon syrup were added to the above solution and mixed well.

4. Sufficient syrup was added to produce the required volume.

Category

Anti- tussive.

Dose

5 ml

Direction

To be sipped and swallowed slowly without adding water.

Storage

Store in a cool and dry place. Protect from light.

Marketed Formulations

CODO- Q (IPCA)

CODYLEX (Anglo French)

EXPERIMENT 13

Paediatric Codeine Linctus BPC

Aim

To prepare and submit 20 ml of Paediatric Codeine Linctus.

Synonym

Codeine Mixture, Paediatric.

Formula

Sl.No	Ingredients	Official formula	Working formula
1	Codeine Linctus	200 ml	
2	Syrup (q.s)	1000ml	

Principle

Paediatric Codeine linctus is used in children as an anti-tussive for the treatment of cough. Children require lower doses than adults. Therefore codeine linctus is diluted with syrup to prepare Paediatric codeine linctus.

Procedure

Codeine linctus and syrup were mixed to form Paediatric Codeine linctus.

Category

Anti-tussive.

Dose

Child – Upto 1 year: 5 ml

1 – 5 years: 10 ml

Direction

To be sipped and swallowed slowly without adding water.

Storage

Store in a cool and dry place. Protect from light.

EXPERIMENT 14

Diabetic
Codeine Linctus BPC

Aim

To prepare and submit 20 ml of Diabetic Codeine Linctus.

Formula

Sl. No	Ingredients	Official formula	Working formula
1	Codeine Phosphate	3 g	
2	Citric acid	5 g	
3	Lemon Spirit	1 ml	
4	Compound Tartrazine solution	10 ml	
5	Benzoic acid solution	20 ml	
6	Chloroform Spirit	20 ml	
7	Purified water	20 ml	
8	Sorbitol solution (q.s)	1000 ml	

Principle

Linctuses are sweetened, viscous liquid preparations usually prescribed for the relief of cough. Linctuses should be sipped and swallowed slowly and should not be diluted before use in order to obtain contact between the drug and mucous membrane of the throat for a longer period of time.

Diabetic Codeine Linctus is usually prescribed for Diabetic patients.

In the following preparation, Codeine Phosphate is an anti-tussive. Lemon syrup is the flavoring agent. Linctuses made with sorbitol solution or syrup support microbial growth and this is prevented by adding Benzoic acid solution and/ or Chloroform spirit as preservatives. Compound tartrazine solution is the colouring agent.

Sorbitol is used as a 70% W/W solution which is about half as sweet as simple syrup. When taken orally, there is no rise in blood sugar and therefore it can be used to replace simple syrup in formulations for diabetics. Like invert syrup, it can be mixed with simple syrup to prevent crystallization on storage.

Procedure

1. Codeine Phosphate and citric acid was dissolved in water.

2. 750 ml of the sorbitol solution was added to it and mixed well.

3. Compound tartrazine solution, benzoic acid solution, chloroform spirit and lemon spirit were added to the above solution and mixed well.

4. Sufficient sorbitol solution was added to produce the required volume.

Category

Anti- tussive.

Dose

5 ml

Direction

To be sipped and swallowed slowly without adding water.

Storage

Store in a cool and dry place. Protect from light.

Solutions

Solutions are liquid preparations that contain one or more chemical substances dissolved in a suitable solvent or mixture of mutually miscible solvents.

Formulation

1. Vehicle - usually purified water.

2. Co-solvents - are employed to increase the solubility of the therapeutic agent in the vehicle. E.g. alcohol, propylene glycol, glycerin.

3. Sweeteners - are used to increase the palatability of the formulation. E.g. sucrose, sorbitol, glucose, saccharin, aspartame.

4. Viscosity enhancers - E.g. hydrophilic polymers such as cellulose derivatives, alginic acid, poly vinyl pyrrolidone.

5. Preservatives - protect the preparation from microbial growth. E.g. p-hydroxybenzoate esters (methyl hydroxybenzoate and propyl hydroxybenzoate), boric acid and borate salts, sorbic acid and sorbate salts.

6. Antioxidants - are included in pharmaceutical solutions to enhance the stability of therapeutic agents that are susceptible to chemical degradation by oxidation E.g. sodium sulphite, sodium metabisulphite, butylated hydroxyanisole (BHA), butylated hydroxytoluene (BHT) and propyl gallate.

   Antioxidants can be used along with chelating agents such as ethylene diamine tetra acetic acid (EDTA) and citric acid to form complexes with heavy-metal ions or ions that are normally involved in oxidative degradation of therapeutic agents.

7. Flavours - The four basic taste sensations are salty, sweet, bitter and sour. It has been proposed that certain flavours should be used to mask these specific taste sensations.

Taste of product	Suitable masking flavour
Salty	Apricot, Butterscotch, Liquorice, Peach, Vanilla and Wintergreen mint
Bitter	Anise, Chocolate, Mint, Passion fruit, Wild cherry
Sweet	Vanilla, Fruits, Berries
Sour	Citrus fruits, Liquorice, Raspberry

8. Colours - the colors used should complement the flavour of the preparation. E.g. green for mint-flavoured solutions, red for strawberry-flavoured formulations, yellow for pineapple flavour, etc.

9. Buffers - are employed to control the pH of the formulated product. The pH controlled to maintain the solubility of the therapeutic agent and to enhance the stability of products. E.g. citrate buffer (citric acid and sodium citrate), acetate buffer (acetic acid and sodium acetate) and phosphate buffer (sodium phosphate and disodium phosphate).

EXPERIMENT 15

Cresol with Soap Solution IP

Aim

To prepare and submit 20 ml of Cresol with Soap solution.

Synonym

Lysol (or) Liquor Cresolis Saponatus.

Formula

Sl.No	Ingredients	Official formula	Working formula
1	Cresol	500 ml	
2	Vegetable oil	180 g	
3	Potassium Hydroxide	42 g	
4	Purified water (q.s)	1000 ml	

Principle

The solubility of cresol in water is upto 2 %v/v but in this preparation, the strength of cresol is 50% v/v. The solubility has been increased by the technique known as **micellar solubilization-** using soap as the solubilizing agent or surfactant. Soap is produced by saponification process, where a vegetable oil is heated with potassium hydroxide to form a monovalent soap.

$$\text{R-COOR}^1 + \text{KOH} \xrightarrow{\text{saponification}} \text{RCOOK} + \text{R}^1\text{-OH}$$

(Unsaturated fatty acid)   (Soap)

Cresol is then solubilized in the soap formed.

Procedure

1. Potassium Hydroxide was dissolved in ¼ the quantity of purified water.
2. The vegetable oil was added and the mixture was heated on a water bath. It was mixed thoroughly and heated continuously until a small portion of the resulting solution dissolves completely in water without the separation of oily drops.
3. Cresol was then added and mixed. Sufficient purified water was added to produce the required volume.

Category

Disinfectant.

Auxiliary label

FOR INANIMATE USE ONLY.

Storage

Store in a cool and dry place away from reach of children.

Protect from light.

EXPERIMENT 16

Aqueous Iodine Solution IP

Aim

To prepare and submit 20 ml of Aqueous Iodine solution.

Synonym

Lugol's solution (or) Liqour Iodi Compositus(or) Liqour Iodi Aquosus.

Formula

Sl.No	Ingredients	Official formula	Working formula
1	Iodine	50 g	
2	Potassium Iodide	100 g	
3	Purified water (q.s)	1000 ml	

Principle

Iodine is sparingly soluble in water. To increase its solubility, Potassium Iodide is added. Iodine combines with Potassium Iodide to form a compound called polyiodide, e.g., $KI.I_2$, $KI.2I_2$, $KI.3I_2$.

The higher polyiodides are more soluble than the lower polyiodides and are formed in concentrated solution. Hence rapid solution of Iodine is achieved by using Potassium iodide in concentrated solution.

Aqueous iodine solution is used as an iodine supplement in goitre which is caused by iodine deficiency.

Procedure

1. Potassium Iodide was dissolved in ¾ the quantity of purified water.
2. Iodine was added to the above solution with continuous stirring till the iodine crystals are completely solubilized.
3. The solution was then made upto the volume with purified water.

Category

Iodine supplement in Goitre.

Dose

5 ml to be taken thrice a day.

Storage

Store in a cool and dark place.

EXPERIMENT 17

Strong Iodine Solution IP

Aim

To prepare and submit 20 ml of Strong Iodine solution.

Synonym

Strong tincture of Iodine (or) Liquor Iodi Fortis.

Formula

Sl.No	Ingredients	Official formula	Working formula
1	Iodine	100 g	
2	Potassium Iodide	60 g	
3	Purified water	100 ml	
4	Alcohol 90% (q.s)	1000 ml	

Principle

Iodine is sparingly soluble in water. To increase its solubility, Potassium Iodide is added. Iodine combines with Potassium Iodide to form a compound called polyiodide, Eg. $KI.I_2$, $KI.2I_2$, $KI.3I_2$.

The higher polyiodides are more soluble than the lower polyiodides and are formed in concentrated solution. Hence rapid solution of Iodine is achieved by using Potassium iodide in concentrated solution.

Alcohol is used as the solvent because it evaporates quickly when the solution is applied on the skin. By dissolving the cutaneous fat, it hastens penetration and absorption. This preparation is used externally as an antiseptic.

Procedure

1. Potassium Iodide was dissolved in ¾ the quantity of purified water.

2. Iodine was added to the above solution with continuous stirring till the iodine crystals were completely solubilized.

3. Remaining water was added. The solution was then made upto volume with alcohol.

Category

Antiseptic.

Auxiliary label

FOR EXTERNAL USE ONLY.

Storage

Store in a cool and dark place.

Marketed Formulations

STRONG IODINE SOLUTION (containing Povidone Iodine)

BETADINE STD SOLUTION (Win Medicare)

MICROSHIELD PVP (Johnson & Johnson)

PIODIN (GSK)

EXPERIMENT 18

Weak Iodine Solution BP

Aim

To prepare and submit 20 ml of Weak Iodine solution.

Synonym

Tincture of Iodine.

Liquor Iodi Mitis.

Formula

Sl.No	Ingredients	Official formula	Working formula
1	Iodine	25 g	
2	Potassium Iodide	25 g	
3	Purified water	25 ml	
4	Alcohol 90% (q.s)	1000 ml	

Principle

Alcohol is used as the solvent because it evaporates quickly when the solution is applied on the skin. By dissolving the cutaneous fat, it hastens penetration and absorption.

Procedure

1. Potassium Iodide and Iodine were dissolved in a small quantity of alcohol.

2. The solution was then made upto volume with the remaining alcohol.

Category

Antiseptic.

Auxiliary label

FOR EXTERNAL USE ONLY.

Storage

Store in a cool and dark place.

48   Pharmaceutics: A Practical Manual

EXPERIMENT 19

Weak Iodine Solution IP

Aim

To prepare and submit 20 ml of Weak Iodine solution.

Synonym

Tincture of Iodine.

Liquor Iodi Mitis.

Formula

Sl.No	Ingredients	Official formula	Working formula
1	Iodine	25 g	
2	Potassium Iodide	25 g	
3	Alcohol 50% (q.s)	1000 ml	

Principle

Alcohol is used as the solvent because it evaporates quickly when the solution is applied on the skin. By dissolving the cutaneous fat, it hastens penetration and absorption.

Procedure

1. Potassium Iodide and Iodine were dissolved in a small quantity of alcohol.

2. The solution was then made upto volume with the remaining alcohol.

Category

Antiseptic.

Auxiliary label

FOR EXTERNAL USE ONLY.

Storage

Store in a cool and dark place.

EXPERIMENT 20

Strong Ammonium Acetate Solution IP

Aim

To prepare and submit 20 ml of strong ammonium acetate solution.

Synonym

Liquor Ammonii Acetatis Fortis.

Formula

Sl.No	Ingredients	Official formula	Working formula
1	Ammonium Bicarbonate	470 g	
2	Glacial acetic acid	453 g	
3	Strong Ammonia Solution	q.s	
4	Purified water (q.s)	1000 ml	

Principle

In this preparation glacial acetic acid reacts with ammonium bicarbonate to form ammonium acetate with the evolution of Carbon dioxide.

$$NH_4HCO_3 + CH_3COOH \longrightarrow CH_3COONH_4 + H_2O + CO_2 \uparrow$$

Ammonium bicarbonate   Ammonium acetate

The excess of acetic acid is neutralized by using strong ammonia solution which forms ammonium acetate and the final pH of the preparation will be between 7.6 – 8.

$$CH_3COOH + NH_4OH \longrightarrow CH_3COONH_4 + H_2O$$
$$\text{Ammonium acetate}$$

Ammonia must be used to complete neutralization because ammonium bicarbonate will not react in the concentrated solution produced above. The final pH is detected by using two indicators – **Bromothymol Blue and Thymol Blue.**

1. Bromothymol Blue gives

$$\begin{array}{ccc} \text{pH 6} & & \text{pH 7.6} \\ \text{Yellow} \longrightarrow \text{green} & \longrightarrow & \text{blue} \end{array}$$

2. Thymol Blue gives

$$\begin{array}{cc} \text{pH 8} & \text{pH 9.6} \\ \text{Yellow} \longrightarrow & \text{blue} \end{array}$$

Hence the neutral pH specified lies between 7.6 and 8.

Procedure

1. Glacial acetic acid was mixed with 350 ml of purified water.
2. Ammonium Bicarbonate was added to the above solution, small quantity at a time with constant stirring until it is completely dissolved. The solution was allowed to stand until effervescence ceases.
3. Sufficient quantity of ammonia solution was added to the above solution until a drop of the resulting solution diluted with ten drops of water gives a full blue colour with one drop of bromothymol blue solution and a full yellow colour with one drop of thymol blue solution.
4. Sufficient water was added to produce the required volume.

Category

Mild Expectorant, Diuretic and Diaphoretic.

Dose

1- 4 ml

Storage

Store in a lead free glass bottle in a cool and dry place. (Because ammonium acetate reacts with lead to give lead acetate, which is toxic).

EXPERIMENT 21

Strong Solution of Ferric Chloride BPC

Aim

To prepare and submit 20 ml of strong solution of ferric chloride.

Synonym

Liquor Ferri Perchloridi Fortis.

Formula

Sl.No	Ingredients	Official formula	Working formula
1	Iron	210 g	
2	Hydrochloric acid	1230 ml	
3	Nitric acid	90 ml	
4	Water (q.s)		

Principle

Iron wire contains carbon, iron carbide etc. so that the portion of iron to be dissolved is controlled by the amount of hydrochloric acid used. Hence an accurate amount of hydrochloric acid with an excess of iron is used.

Strong solution of ferric chloride is prepared as follows.

1. Preparation of ferrous chloride by heating iron wire & hydrochloric acid until hydrogen ceases to be evolved. That is until al hydrochloric acid has been used.

$$Fe + 2HCl \longrightarrow FeCl_2 + H_2 \uparrow$$
$$\text{Ferrous chloride}$$

This solution is then filtered to remove iron carbide etc. & the flask is washed with water so that the filtrate contains all the ferrous chloride that is formed.

2. The next stage consists of oxidizing the ferrous chloride to ferrichloride. The reaction necessitates the presence of more hydrochloric acid to supply the chlorine irons necessary for the formation of ferric chloride.

$$2FeCl_2 + Cl_2 \longrightarrow 2FeCl_3$$
$$\text{Ferric chloride}$$

Nitric acid is used as the oxidizing agent because its reduction products are volatile and can be removed by boiling. Hence the ferrous chloride solution is mixed with hydrochloric acid and poured into nitric acid and heated.

Reactions may be represented as-

$$2HNO_3 \longrightarrow H_2O + N_2O_5$$
$$N_2O_5 \longrightarrow 2NO + 3\,O$$
$$6HCl + 3O \longrightarrow 3H_2O + 3\,Cl_2$$
$$6FeCl_2 + 3Cl_2 \longrightarrow 6FeCl_3$$

or written as a combined equation

$$3FeCl_2 + 3\,HCl + HNO_3 \longrightarrow 3FeCl_3 + 2H_2O + NO$$

3. The liquid is then evaporated until precipitation of ferric oxychloride commences, due to hydrolysis.

$$FeCl_3 + H_2O \longrightarrow Fe\,(OH)Cl_2 + HCl$$

The precipitate is not easily recognized until an appreciable quantity has been formed. The pungent fumes of hydrochloric acid are more easily recognized and detection of the evolution of hydrochloric acid is better indication of when to stop evaporation.

4. A specified quantity of hydrochloric acid is then added so that the precipitate of ferric oxychloride dissolves. The above reaction proceeds from right to left. This solution could now be subjected to analysis and diluted with distilled water to form a solution of ferric chloride.

Procedure

1. Iron was placed in a flask. A mixture of 750 ml of hydrochloric acid and 420ml of water was added. It was then heated at a moderate temperature until effervescence ceases.
2. The mixture was boiled and filtered from undissolved iron.
3. The flask was washed with a little water and the washings are poured over the filter.
4. To the combined filtrate & washings, 420 ml of hydrochloric acid was added and mixed.
5. This solution was then poured in a thin stream into nitric acid, chemical action been promoted, if necessary by gentle warming.
6. The product was evaporated until a precipitate was formed.
7. 60 ml of hydrochloric acid and sufficient water was added to produce 1050 ml.

Category

Astringent (used as a styptic to arrest bleeding from small wounds).

Auxiliary label

FOR EXTERNAL USE ONLY.

Storage

Store in a cool and dry place.

Surgical Chlorinated Soda Solution BPC

Aim

To prepare and submit 20 ml of Surgical Chlorinated Soda solution BPC.

Synonym

Dakin's solution; Liquor Sodae Chlorinatae Chirurgicalis.

Formula

Sl. No	Ingredients	Official formula	Working formula
1	Boric Acid	q.s	
2	Chlorinated Lime	q.s	
3	Sodium carbonate	q.s	
4	Purified water(q.s)	1000 ml	

Principle

Dakin's solution is used by continuous irrigation to clean infected wounds and burns. It must be applied every two hours. The solution is irritating to the surrounding skin, which should be protected by lining with petroleum jelly. It is also applied as a lotion or wet dressing for superficial wounds and burns. Suitably diluted Dakin's solution can also be used as a gargle for the treatment of tonsillitis, as an irrigation solution for infections of bladder and vagina. It can also used as a foot bath for the prophylaxis of fungal infections of the feet.

The preparation involves the determination of available chlorine in the sample of chlorinated lime (bleaching powder) that is to be used in the preparation. From this the required amounts of chlorinated lime, sodium carbonate and boric acid can be calculated.

The content of available chlorine can be assayed by the following method:

Triturate 4 g of chlorinated lime, with successive small portions of water. The combined triturates are then diluted to 1000 ml with water and mixed thoroughly. 100 ml of this suspension is then mixed with a solution containing 3 g of potassium iodide in 100ml of water. 5ml of acetic acid is then added to this mixture. The liberated iodine is titrated with 0.1N sodium thiosulphate. Each ml of 0.1N sodium thiosulphate is equivalent to 0.003545g of chlorine.

The content of chlorine should be not less than 30%.

Avaialable chlorine in chlorinated lime %	Chlorinated Lime(g)	Sodium Carbonate (g)	Boric acid(g)
30	18.8	37.6	4.00
31	18.2	36.4	3.87
32	17.6	35.2	3.75
33	17.1	34.2	3.64
34	16.6	33.2	3.53
35	16.1	32.2	3.43
36	15.7	31.4	3.33
37	15.3	30.6	3.24
38	14.9	29.8	3.16
39	14.5	29.0	3.08
40	14.1	28.2	3.00

Calcium chlorohypochlorite, the main constituent of bleaching powder, is decomposed by water.

$$2\ Ca(OCl)Cl \longrightarrow Ca(OCl)_2 + CaCl_2$$
$$\text{Calcium hypochlorite}$$

The calcium hypochlorite and calcium chloride react with the sodium carbonate.

$$Ca(OCl)_2 + Na_2CO_3 \longrightarrow 2NaOCl + CaCO_3$$
$$\text{Sodium hypochlorite}$$

$$CaCl_2 + Na_2CO_3 \longrightarrow 2NaCl + CaCO_3$$

The filtrate contains sodium hypochlorite and sodium chloride.

Bleaching powder always contains some calcium hydroxide which also reacts with the sodium carbonate.

$$Ca(OH)_2 + Na_2CO_3 \longrightarrow 2NaOH + CaCO_3$$

Sodium hypochlorite also undergoes hydrolysis in solution to produce sodium hydroxide.

$$NaOCl + H_2O \longrightarrow NaOH + HOCl$$

The last two reactions make the filtrate very alkaline and too caustic for wound treatment. Hence Boric acid is added to neutralize the sodium hydroxide and buffer the pH at about 9.5.

$$2NaOH + 4H_3BO_3 \longrightarrow Na_2B_4O_7 + 7H_2O$$

Sodium hypochlorite solutions are most stable at alkaline pH. Hence this preparation is a compromise between irritancy and stability.

The preparation retains its potency for 3 to 4 weeks when stored in well closed, light resistant containers in a cool place.

Procedure

1. Sodium carbonate was dissolved in water.
2. The above solution was added slowly to powdered chlorinated lime, with continuous trituration.
3. The solution was shaken occasionally during twenty minutes, allowed to stand for a further 10 minutes, decanted and filtered through a bleached filter paper. (The solution bleaches grey filter paper, turning the filtrate yellow and reducing its strength).
4. Boric acid was then dissolved in the filtrate.

Category

Antiseptic.

Auxiliary label

FOR EXTERNAL USE ONLY.

Storage

Store in a well-closed container in a cool and dry place.

Protect from light.

EXPERIMENT 23

Chloroxylenol Solution BPC

Aim

To prepare and submit 20 ml of Chloroxylenol Solution I.P.

Synonym

Roxenol ;Liquor Chloroxylenolis.

Formula

Sl. No	Ingredients	Official formula	Working formula
1	Castor oil	63 g	
2	Chloroxylenol	50g	
3	Potassium Hydroxide	13.6 g	
4	Alcohol (95%)	200 ml	
5	Terpineol	100 ml	
6	Oleic acid	7.5 ml	
7	Purified water (q.s)	1000 ml	

Principle

Chloroxylenol solution is an antiseptic solution used in surgical and obstetrical practice and to maintain hygiene at home. It is also used for cuts, wounds and abrasions.

Chloroxylenol is only slightly soluble in water (1 in 3000); hence in this preparation soap is used to increase its solubility. Chloroxylenol solution is a clear colloidal solution in which chloroxylenol is solubilized by the soap micelles. On dilution with water a fine white solution is produced.

Castor oil soap, consisting mainly of potassium ricinoleate, is made by saponification process. The process involves dissolving potassium hydroxide in a little water, adding a solution of castor oil in 95% alcohol, mixing and setting aside for about an hour until a small portion gives a clear solution with 19 times its volume of water. Saponification occurs more quickly in alcoholic solution and therefore it is important not to exceed the volume of water used for dissolving the alkali. The soap solution solubilizes the chloroxylenol and acts as an emulsifying agent when the solution is diluted.

Oleic acid is added to the soap to neutralize excess alkali and to give a pH of optimum bactericidal effect. This is necessary because the germicidal action of Chloroxylenol is reduced in alkaline solutions.

Chloroxylenol and terpineol are only slightly soluble in water but very soluble in alcohol (95%). Chloroxylenol is readily soluble in terpineol. The Terpineol helps to prevent separation of Chloroxylenol on dilution and contributes to the characteristic odour of the preparation.

Procedure

1. Potassium Hydroxide was dissolved in 15 ml of water.
2. Castor oil was added to 63 ml of alcohol.
3. The castor oil solution was then mixed with the potassium hydroxide solution and allowed to stand for one hour or until a small portion of the mixture remains clear when diluted with nineteen times its volume of purified water. The soap solution formed was kept aside.
4. Oleic acid was then added until a few drops of the soap solution gave a bluish green colour with bromothymol blue solution.
5. Chloroxylenol was mixed with the remaining alcohol and terpineol was added to it.
6. The above solution was then added to the soap solution, with stirring.
7. Sufficient water was added to produce the required volume.

Category

Antiseptic (Germicide) – in First aid, Medical and Personal hygiene.

Auxiliary label

FOR EXTERNAL USE ONLY.

Storage

Store in a cool and dry place.

Marketed Formulation

DETTOL Antiseptic Liquid (Reckitt Benckiser).

EXPERIMENT 24

Sodium Chloride Solution IP

Aim

To prepare and submit 20 ml of Sodium Chloride solution I.P.

Synonym

Normal saline.

Formula

Sl. No	Ingredients	Official formula	Working formula
1	Sodium Chloride	9 g	
2	Purified water (q.s)	1000 ml	

Principle

Sodium chloride is mainly used as a tonicity adjusting agent, fluid and electrolyte repelenisher.

If sodium chloride solution is to be used for injection, then purified water has to be replaced by Water for Injection.

E.g. Sodium Chloride injection IP is a sterile 0.9% W/V solution of Sodium Chloride in Water for Injection. It contains no antimicrobial agent.

Procedure

Sodium Chloride was dissolved in purified water and filtered.

Category

Tonicity adjusting agent.

Storage

Store in a wellclosed container in a cool and dry place.

Liniments

Liniments are alcoholic or oleaginous solutions or emulsions of various medicinal substances intended to be rubbed on the skin. Liniments with an alcoholic or hydroalcoholic vehicle are useful when rubefacient, counterirritant or penetrating action is desired. Oleaginous liniments are employed when massage is desired. They are less irritating to the skin than alcoholic liniments.

Liniments should be applied on to the skin with rubbing and should never be applied on the broken parts of the skin. Since they are rubbed onto the affected area, liniments are also called as embrocations.

The vehicle for the liniment should be selected on the basis of the solubility of the ingredients in solvents and depending on the type of action required- rubefacient, counter irritant or massage. For oleaginous liniments, the vehicle may be a fixed oil such as almond oil, peanut oil, sesame oil or cottonseed oil or a volatile oil such as wintergreen oil or turpentine oil or it may be a combination of fixed and volatile oils.

Direction for Usage

To be applied on the skin with friction.

Label

For external use only.

Not to be applied on cut or broken skin.

Shake well before use.

Keep out of reach of children.

Containers

Liniments are supplied in coloured fluted bottles to distinguish them from preparations meant for internal use.

Marketed Formulations

ARTHRILL (Ind-Swift)

MYOSTAL LINIMENT

SLOANS LINIMENT (Lee Pharmaceuticals)

EXPERIMENT 25

Turpentine Liniment IP

Aim

To prepare and submit 20 ml of Turpentine liniment.

Synonym

Linimentum Terebinthinae.

Formula

Sl.No	Ingredients	Official formula	Working formula
1	Turpentine oil	650 ml	
2	Soft-soap	90 g	
3	Camphor	50 g	
4	Purified water (q.s)	1000 ml	

Principle

Liniments are liquid or semi solid preparations meant for application on to the skin. They are usually applied with friction and rubbing of the skin. A liniment should not be applied to the broken skin because it may cause excessive irritation.

Turpentine liniment is an emulsion type liniment made with alkali soap. It is an O/W emulsion prepared using soft soap as the emulsifying agent. Turpentine oil with camphor acts as the dispersed phase and the continuous phase is the soap solution (soft soap and water).

Procedure

1. Soft soap was mixed with 100 ml of purified water.
2. Camphor was dissolved in turpentine oil.
3. The camphor mixture was then slowly added to the soap mixture with trituration until a thick creamy emulsion was formed.
4. Sufficient water was added to produce the required volume and mixed.

Category

Counter irritant and rubefacient.

Direction

To be applied on the skin with friction.

Auxiliary label

FOR EXTERNAL USE ONLY.

NOT TO BE APPLIED ON BROKEN SKIN.

SHAKE WELL BEFORE USE.

Storage

Store in a cool and dry place.

EXPERIMENT 26

Camphor Liniment

Aim

To prepare and submit 20 ml of Camphor liniment.

Synonym

Camphorated oil.

Linimentum Camphorae.

Formula

Sl.No	Ingredients	Standard formula	Working formula
1	Camphor	200 g	
2	Arachis oil	800 g	

Principle

Camphor acts as a counter irritant and anti-pruritic. Arachis oil is the base and provides easy application and massaging. It is also less irritant when compared to alcohol.

Since liniments are applied on the restricted topical areas with massage, their preparations must be highly viscous.

Procedure

Camphor was dissolved in the arachis oil in a closed vessel.

Category

Counter irritant and anti-pruritic.

Direction

To be applied on the skin with friction.

Auxiliary label

FOR EXTERNAL USE ONLY.

NOT TO BE APPLIED ON BROKEN SKIN.

SHAKE WELL BEFORE USE.

Storage

Store in a cool and dry place away from light.

Soap Liniment BP

Aim

To prepare and submit 20 ml of Soap liniment.

Synonym

Linimentum Saponis.

Formula

Sl.No	Ingredients	Official formula	Working formula
1	Soft soap	80 g	
2	Camphor	40 g	
3	Rosemary oil	15 ml	
4	Distilled water	170 ml	
5	Alcohol 90% (q.s)	1000 ml	

Principle

Soap liniment is a mild counter irritant used in the treatment of sprains and bruises.

Camphor is a counter irritant and antipruritic. Rosemary oil is used topically, to treat muscle pain and arthritis and to improve circulation

Procedure

1. Soft soap, camphor and rosemary oil was dissolved in ¾ the volume of alcohol.
2. Distilled water was added to it and set aside for 7 days.
3. The solution was then filtered and made upto volume with alcohol.

Category

Counter irritant and rubefacient.

Direction

To be applied on the skin with friction.

Auxiliary label

FOR EXTERNAL USE ONLY.

NOT TO BE APPLIED ON BROKEN SKIN.

SHAKE WELL BEFORE USE.

Storage

Store in a cool and dry place away from light.

Keep away from naked flame.

Suspensions

Suspensions are biphasic; heterogenous systems in which finely divided insoluble solid particles (disperse phase) are dispersed or suspended in a vehicle (dispersion medium). The diameter of the disperse phase may range from 0.5 to 100 μm. Systems in which the particle size diameter falls below the above range are termed colloidal.

A suspension would be considered stable if, after agitation (shaking), the drug particles are homogeneously dispersed for a sufficient time to ensure that an accurate dose is removed for administration to the patient.

Properties of a Good Suspension

1. The dispersed particles should settle slowly and should redisperse immediately on shaking.

2. The product should remain sufficiently homogenous for at least the period between shaking the container and removing the required dose.

3. The viscosity of the suspension should be such that it can be easily removed from the container and transferred to the site of application without any difficulty.

4. The sediment produced on standing should not form a hard cake.

5. Any suspended particles should be small and uniformly sized in order to give a smooth, elegant shaped particle, free from grittiness.

6. The suspension should be chemically stable.

Diffusible Suspensions

These are suspensions containing light powders which are insoluble, or only very slightly soluble in the vehicle, but which on shaking disperse evenly throughout the vehicle for long enough to allow an accurate dose to be withdrawn.

Indiffusible Suspensions

These are suspensions containing heavy powders which are insoluble in the vehicle and which on shaking do not disperse evenly throughout the vehicle long enough to allow an accurate dose to be withdrawn. Indiffusible suspensions contain a suspending agent or a thickening agent to slow the rate at which the powder settles.

Sl.No	Flocculated suspension	Deflocculated suspension
1	Particles form loose aggregates or network like structure called floccules.	Particles exist as separate entities.
2	Rate of sedimentation is high	Rate of sedimentation is less.
3	Sediment is loosely packed and does not form a hard cake.	Sediment is closely packed and forma a hard cake.
4	Sediment is easy to redisperse	Sediment is difficult to redisperse
5	The supernatant liquid becomes clear very quickly	Supernatant liquid will remain cloudy for a long time due to slow settling of particles.
6	Product will not be pleasing in appearance	Product will be pleasing in appearance

Formulation of Suspensions

1. Medicament
2. *Flocculating agents:* E.g. Surfactants , electrolytes
3. *Suspending agents:* E.g. bentonite
4. *Thickening agents:* E.g. Acacia. Tragacanth, Sodium CMC, Methyl cellulose
5. *Wetting agents:* E.g. Spans and Tweens
6. *Preservatives:* E.g. benzoic acid, methyl and propyl paraben
7. Organoleptic additives

    - *Flavouring agents:* E.g. vanilla flavour, banana flavour, strawberry flavour
    - *Sweetening agents:* E.g. Sucrose, Saccharin sodium, aspartame
    - *Colouring agents:* E.g. amaranth, tartrazine

Choice of Suspending Agent

The amount of suspending agent used in any given formulation depends on the volume of vehicle being thickened. It does not vary with the amount of powder in the preparation. A suspending agent is intended to increase the viscosity of the vehicle and therefore slow down sedimentation rates. This outcome could also be achieved by decreasing the particle size of the powder in suspension.

The most common suspending agents used in extemporaneous dispensing are Tragacanth BP (internal or external suspensions), Compound Tragacanth Powder BP (containing: 15% Tragacanth BP, 20% Acacia BP, 20% Starch BP and 45% Sucrose BP) (internal suspensions) and Bentonite BP (external suspensions).

Auxiliary Label

SHAKE WELL BEFORE USE.

EXPERIMENT 28

Calamine Lotion IP

Aim

To prepare and submit 20 ml of calamine lotion.

Synonym

Lotio calamine.

Formula

Sl. No	Ingredients	Official formula	Working formula
1	Calamine	150 g	
2	Zinc Oxide	50 g	
3	Bentonite	30 g	
4	Sodium citrate	5 g	
5	Glycerin	50 ml	
6	Liquified Phenol	5 ml	
7	Rose water (q.s)	1000 ml	

Principle

Lotions are usually suspensions or dispersions intended for external application. Calamine is chemically a mixture of zinc oxide and small amounts of ferric oxide. It is light pink in colour and matches well with the colour of the skin.

Calamine and Zinc oxide have protective and astringent properties. Zinc oxide and calamine are indiffusible solids; therefore Bentonite (colloidal hydrated aluminum silicate - inorganic clay) is added as the suspending agent. But Bentonite causes marked flocculation and makes the preparation difficult to pour. Therefore Sodium citrate is included to produce partial deflocculation and thus makes the preparation pourable. It also acts as a buffer and prevents the oxidation of ferric oxide.

Glycerin is a humectant. Liquified Phenol is the preservative. Rose water is used as the vehicle and as the perfume to mask the phenolic odour of liquefied phenol.

Procedure

1. Sodium citrate was dissolved in 700 ml of Rose water.
2. Calamine, Zinc oxide and Bentonite were triturated with the sodium citrate solution.
3. Liquified phenol and glycerin were added to the suspension and made upto volume with rose water.

Category

Protective, astringent, soothing agent and skin tonic.

Auxiliary label

FOR EXTERNAL USE ONLY.

SHAKE WELL BEFORE USE.

Storage

Store in a well-closed container in a cool and dry place.

Marketed Formulations

LACTOCALAMINE (Nicholas Piramal)

CALADRYL (Pfizer)

CALAK LOTION (SPPL)

CIMFI (Aamorb)

CALASOFT LOTION (Microgratia)

EXPERIMENT 29

Magnesium Hydroxide Mixture BP

Aim

To prepare and submit 20 ml of Magnesium Hydroxide mixture.

Synonym

Cream of Magnesia.

Milk of Magnesia.

Formula

Sl. No	Ingredients	Official formula	Working formula
1	Light Magnesium Oxide	52.5 g	
2	Magnesium Sulphate	47.5 g	
3	Sodium Hydroxide	15 g	
4	Chloroform	2.5 ml	
5	Purified water (q.s)	1000 ml	

Principle

Milk of magnesia is an aqueous colloidal dispersion of magnesium hydroxide, which can be prepared by 2 methods.

(Colloidal dispersions are disperse systems whose particle are of the size range 1nm – 0.5μm).

Precipitation method: In this method, Sodium hydroxide reacts with Magnesium Sulphate to form a precipitate of magnesium hydroxide and sodium sulphate. The precipitate obtained will sediment quickly.

$$MgSO_4 + 2NaOH \longrightarrow Mg(OH)_2 \downarrow \; + Na_2SO_4$$

Hydration method: Magnesium hydroxide is prepared by the hydration of light magnesium oxide. The hydration requires 48 hrs for completion and the magnesium hydroxide formed will be very viscous and unpourable.

$$MgO + H_2O \longrightarrow Mg(OH)_2 \downarrow$$

Therefore magnesium hydroxide mixture is prepared by a combination of precipitation and hydration methods in order to give a precipitate that is not thick and does not sediment rapidly.

Dilute solutions should be used in order to obtain a fine precipitate of magnesium hydroxide.

Chloroform is used as a preservative.

The precipitate should be washed till is free from sulphate, which can be tested using Barium Chloride solution. This is done because the sodium sulphate formed by the precipitation reaction, if left behind in the preparation acts as a purgative.

Test for sulphates

To a small quantity of the washings, add 0.5M Barium Chloride solution. Any turbidity produced indicates the presence of sulphates.

$$BaCl_2 + Na_2SO_4 \longrightarrow BaSO_4 \downarrow + 2NaCl$$

Procedure

1. Sodium Hydroxide was dissolved in 150 ml of water.

2. Light Magnesium Oxide was triturated with this solution to form a smooth cream. Sufficient water was added to produce 250 ml.

3. This suspension was then poured in a thin stream into a solution of magnesium sulphate in 250 ml of water, stirring continuously. The precipitate was allowed to settle.

4. The supernatant liquid was decanted and the precipitate was washed with water until the washings were free from sulphates.

5. The washed precipitate was then mixed with sufficient water, chloroform was added and the volume was made up.

Category

Antacid and laxative.

Dosage

Antacid - 5 to 10 ml

Laxative – 15 to 30 ml

Auxiliary label

SHAKE WELL BEFORE USE.

Storage

Store in a well-closed container in a cool and dry place.

(This preparation is best stored in tight containers preferably at a temperature above 0°C and below 35°C. Freezing results in coarsening of the disperse phase. (i.e. aggregation of the particles) and the preparation will have a granular appearance. Temperature above 35°C decreases the gel structure).

Note

1. Many commercial preparations contain a combination of aluminium and magnesium compounds. Magnesium salts increase intestinal motility whereas aluminium decreases it. Thus antacids containing magnesium salts tend to be laxative in action and those containing aluminium salts may be constipating. Therefore many commercial preparations contain the right balance of aluminium and magnesium compounds so as not to significantly change bowel function.

2. The pH of magnesium hydroxide mixture is about 10 and therefore attacks lime soda glass containers and imparts a bitter taste to the preparation. The USP which contains a similar preparation, allows inclusion of 0.1% of citric acid to minimize this effect. This concentration of citric acid also improves the flavour of mixtures prepared by hydration alone (which tend to have an alkaline taste).

Marketed Formulations

DEY'S MILK OF MAGNESIA (Dey's)

DIGENE GEL (Abbott)

GELUPIN-MPS (Lupin)

GELUSIL-MPS (Pfizer)

EXPERIMENT 30

Aluminium Hydroxide Gel

Aim

To prepare and submit 20 ml of Aluminium hydroxide gel.

Formula

Sl. No	Ingredients	Official formula	Working formula
1	Aluminum hydroxide (gelatinous)	6 g	
2	Sorbitol	1.4 g	
3	Saccharin Sodium	0.005 g	
4	Peppermint oil	0.005 ml	
5	Sodium benzoate	0.5 g	
6	Purified water (q.s)	100 ml	

Principle

Antacids are over-the-counter medications that help neutralize stomach acid. Aluminium Hydroxide gel is an aqueous suspension of hydrated aluminium oxide together with varying quantities of basic Aluminium carbonate and bicarbonate.

Sorbitol is a stabilizing agent and prevents thickening and hardening of the suspension. Sodium benzoate is the preservative. Saccharin sodium is the sweetener and Peppermint oil is the flavouring agent.

Procedure

1. Aluminium hydroxide was dispersed in water.

2. Sorbitol, Sodium benzoate and Saccharin sodium were added to the dispersion and mixed well.

3. Peppermint oil was added.

4. Sufficient water was added to make up the required volume.

Category

Antacid – helps relieve acid indigestion and heart burn.

Dosage

As directed by the physician.

Auxiliary label

SHAKE WELL BEFORE USE.

DO NOT TAKE MORE THAN 8 TEASPOONFUL IN 24 HOURS OR USE THE MAXIMUM DOSAGE FOR MORE THAN 2 WEEKS.

Storage

Store in a cool and dry place.

(Note: Many commercial preparations contain a combination of aluminium and magnesium compounds. Magnesium salts increase intestinal motility whereas aluminium decreases it. Thus antacids containing magnesium salts tend to be laxative in action and those containing aluminium salts may be constipating. Therefore many commercial preparations contain the right balance of aluminium and magnesium compounds so as not to significantly change bowel function).

Marketed Formulations

ALTERNAGEL

EXPERIMENT 31

Magnesium Trisilicate Mixture BPC

Aim

To prepare and submit 20 ml of Magnesium Trisilicate Mixture.

Synonym

Compound Magnesium Trisilicate Mixture.

Formula

Sl. No	Ingredients	Official formula	Working formula
1	Light Magnesium Carbonate	50 g	
2	Magnesium Trisilicate	50 g	
3	Sodium Bicarbonate	50 g	
4	Peppermint water (q.s)	1000 ml	

Principle

Magnesium Trisilicate mixture is a suspension of diffusible solids. It is used as an antacid. When taken orally, magnesium Trisilicate gets converted to a gel in the stomach, forming a protective and soothing coating over the inflamed mucosa.

Procedure

1. Light magnesium carbonate, Magnesium Trisilicate and sodium bicarbonate are finely powdered, separately.

2. Light magnesium carbonate and Magnesium Trisilicate are then mixed in a mortar.

3. Enough peppermint water was added to the powders to make a smooth paste.

4. Sodium bicarbonate was dissolved in a small portion of peppermint water and added slowly to the paste of powders.

5. The mixture was then diluted with the vehicle until it became pourable and filtered.

6. Pepperrmint water was added to produce the required volume.

Category

Antacid.

Dose

10 – 20 ml.

Auxiliary label

SHAKE WELL BEFORE USE.

Storage

Store in a wellclosed container in a cool and dry place.

EXPERIMENT 32

Paediatric Chalk Mixture BPC

Aim

To prepare and submit 20 ml of Paediatric Chalk Mixture.

Synonym

Mistura Cretae pro Infantibus.

Formula

Sl. No	Ingredients	Official formula	Working formula
1	Chalk	20 g	
2	Tragacanth, powder	2 g	
3	Syrup	100 ml	
4	Concentrated Cinnamon water	4 ml	
5	Chloroform water, double strength	500 ml	
6	Purified water (q.s)	1000 ml	

Principle

Chalk mixture is a suspension of indiffusible solid for oral use, with tragacanth mucilage as suspending agent.

Paediatric chalk mixture is used in the treatment of diarrhoea to absorb toxins from the intestine.

Procedure

1. Tragacanth was triturated with water to form mucilage.
2. The chalk powder was then triturated with the mucilage to form a smooth cream.
3. Syrup and concentrated cinnamon water were added and trituration continued.
4. Chloroform water was added to the mixture to make it pourable.
5. Purified water was added to produce the required volume.

Category

Used in the treatment of diarrhoea to absorb toxins from the intestine.

Dose

Child: Upto 1 year: 5 ml

1 to 5 years: 10 ml

Auxiliary label

SHAKE WELL BEFORE USE.

Storage

Store in a well-closed container in a cool and dry place.

EXPERIMENT 33

Zinc Sulphide Lotion BPC

Aim

To prepare and submit 20 ml Zinc Sulphide Lotion.

Synonym

Sulphurated Potash and Zinc lotion.

Sulphurated Potash lotion.

Formula

Sl. No	Ingredients	Official formula	Working formula
1	Sulphurated Potash	5 g	
2	Zinc Sulphate	5g	
3	Concentrated Camphor water	2.5 ml	
4	Purified water (q.s)	100 ml	

Principle

Zinc Sulphide lotion is a suspension produced by chemical reaction. Here the insoluble active constituent (zinc sulphide) of the lotion is formed by a chemical reaction.

Sulphurated potash is a mixture of potassium polysulphides and other sulphur containing potassium compounds. It should be freshly prepared because the solubility of zinc sulphide decreases on storage.

Sulphurated potash reacts with Zinc sulphate to produce a precipitate of zinc sulphide that is diffusible in nature only if the sulphurated   potash is added to Zinc Sulphate.

If the Zinc Sulphate is added to sulphurated potash, then the precipitate formed will be indiffusible in nature.

A fine precipitate is obtained if dilute solutions of the reactants are mixed. Hence the reacting substances should be dissolved separately in approximately half the volume of the vehicle and the two parts mixed. If the suspension is prepared in this manner, the precipitate will be diffusible and no suspending agent is necessary.

Procedure

1. Sulphurated potash was dissolved in 50 ml water.
2. Zinc Sulphate was also dissolved in 50 ml water.
3. Sulphurated potash solution was added slowly to the Zinc Sulphate solution with constant stirring.
4. Camphor water was added in small amounts with vigorous shaking to redissolve the precipitated camphor.
5. The suspension was made upto volume and mixed.

Category

Used in the treatment of acne and scabies.

Direction

To be applied on the skin with cotton.

Auxiliary label

SHAKE WELL BEFORE USE.

FOR EXTERNAL USE ONLY.

Storage

Store in a cool and dry place.

Emulsions

Emulsions are biphasic heterogeneous systems consisting of two immiscible phases one of which is finely subdivided and distributed as droplets throughout the other. An emulsion is rendered homogeneous by the addition of an emulsifying agent. The emulsifying agent ensures that the droplets (dispersed phase) is finely dispersed throughout the dispersion medium as minute globules.

There are two principal types of emulsion:

1. **Oil in Water (O/W) emulsions**: the oil (internal or dispersed) phase is dispersed as droplets through the aqueous phase (external / continuous phase/dispersion medium). Oil is the dispersed phase and water is the dispersion medium.

2. **Water in Oil (W/O) emulsions**: the internal phase is composed of water droplets and the external phase is non-aqueous. Water is the dispersed phase and oil is the dispersion medium. Generally all oral emulsions tend to be oil-in-water as the oily phase is usually less pleasant to take and more difficult to flavour.

The major use of emulsions is as cream formulations (for external application). However, emulsions may also be administered intravenously, rectally or orally.

Emulsions are physically unstable and the various excipients in the formulation are present primarily to stabilize the physical properties of the system.

Tests for Identification of Emulsions

1. Dilution test
2. Dye solubility test
3. Conductivity test
4. Cobalt chloride test
5. Fluorescence test

Formulation of Emulsions

1. *Vehicle:* Freshly boiled and cooled purified water is normally used because of the increased risk from microbial contamination.
2. Preservative.
3. Emulsifying agent (emulgent): The quantity of emulsifying agent added is determined by the type of oil to be emulsified and the quantity of emulsion to be prepared.
4. Flavouring agent.
5. Colouring agent.

Preparation of Emulsions

The preparation of an emulsion involves two stages:

1. Preparation of the primary emulsion.
2. Dilution of the primary emulsion.

Calculation of Primary Emulsion Formula

The amount of emulsifying agent used is dependent on the amount and type of oil to be emulsified. Oils can be divided into three categories: fixed oils, mineral oils and volatile oils. The ratio of oil to water to gum for a primary emulsion can be calculated using the following formulae:

Type of oil	Examples	Oil	Water	Gum
Fixed oil	Arachis oil, Castor oil, Cod liver oil	4	2	1
Mineral oil	Liquid Paraffin	3	2	1
Volatile (aromatic) oil	Cinnamon oil, Turpentine oil, Peppermint oil	2	2	1
Oleo resin	Male fern extract	1	2	1

These proportions are important when making the primary emulsion, to prevent the emulsion breaking down on dilution or storage.

There are two methods used in the preparation of emulsions:

1. ***Trituration method:*** This includes the dry gum and wet gum method.

   Dry Gum or Continental method: In this method the emulsifying agent (usually acacia) is mixed with the oil before the addition of water.

The acacia is triturated with the oil in a perfectly dry porcelain mortar until thoroughly mixed. A mortar with a rough surface must be used to ensure proper grinding action and reduction of globule size. After the oil and gum have been mixed, the amount of water required for the primary emulsion is added in small portions with continuous trituration. Trituration is continued until the primary emulsion is creamy white and a cracking sound is produced to the movement of the pestle. Other soluble liquid ingredients are then mixed into the primary emulsion. Solid substances such as preservatives, stabilizers, colourants and any flavouring agents are usually dissolved in a suitable volume of vehicle and added to the primary emulsion.

The emulsion is then made upto volume with the remaining vehicle.

Wet Gum or English method: In this method the emulsifying agent is added to the water to form a mucilage and then the oil is slowly incorporated to form the emulsion.

In the wet gum method, the same proportions of oil, water and gum as given in the above table are used, but the order of mixing is different. Mucilage of the gum is prepared by triturating with water. The oil is then added in small portions with trituration. After all of the oil has been added, the mixture is thoroughly triturated to form the primary emulsion. Other soluble liquid ingredients are then mixed into the primary emulsion. Solid substances such as preservatives, stabilizers, colourants and any flavouring agents are usually dissolved in a suitable volume of vehicle and added to the primary emulsion. The emulsion is then made upto volume with the remaining vehicle.

2. ***Bottle or Forbes method:*** This method is employed for preparing emulsions containing volatile and other non-viscous oils. Both dry gum and wet gum methods can be employed for the preparation.

As volatile oils have a low viscosity as compared to fixed oils, they require comparatively large quantity of gum for emulsification. In this method, oil or water is first shaken vigorously with the calculated amount of gum. Once this has emulsified completely, the second liquid (either oil or water) is then added all at once and the bottle is again shaken vigorously to form the primary emulsion. More of water is added in small portions with constant shaking after each addition to produce the final volume.

This method is not suitable for viscous oils as they cannot be thoroughly agitated in the bottle when mixed with the emulgent. When the intended dispersed phase is a mixture of fixed oil and volatile oil, the dry gum is generally employed.

Preparation of Emulsion by Dry Gum Method

Preparation of the primary emulsion

1. The oil is accurately measured in a dry measuring cylinder and transferred into a dry porcelain mortar.

2. The calculated quantity of emulsifying agent is also added to the oil in the mortar, and triturated rapidly to form a uniform mixture.

4. The quantity of water required for the primary emulsion is added and triturated vigorously in a single direction till a clicking sound is produced and a thick creamy emulsion is formed. This is the primary emulsion.

5. The product should be a thick, white cream. Increased degree of whiteness indicates a better-quality product. Oil globules should not be apparent.

Dilution of the primary emulsion

1. The primary emulsion is diluted with very small volumes of the remaining aqueous vehicle. Mixing should be carefully carried out with the pestle in one direction.

2. Other liquid ingredients if present are added and the emulsion is made upto volume.

Preparation of Emulsion by Wet Gum Method

Preparation of the primary emulsion

1. The calculated amount of emulsifying agent is transferred into a dry porcelain mortar.

2. The measured quantity of water is added to the mortar and triturated rapidly to form a uniform mixture.

3. The quantity of oil required for the primary emulsion is added and triturated vigorously in a single direction till a clicking sound is produced and a thick creamy emulsion is formed. This is the primary emulsion.

Dilution of the primary emulsion

1. The primary emulsion is diluted with very small volumes of the remaining aqueous vehicle. Mixing should be carefully carried out with the pestle in one direction.
2. Other liquid ingredients if present are added and the emulsion is made upto volume.

Instabilities in Emulsions

Emulsions can break down in the following ways:

1. Cracking,
2. Creaming,
3. Phase inversion.

Cracking

This is the term applied when the globules of the disperse phase coalesce and forms a separate layer. Redispersion cannot be achieved by shaking and the preparation is no longer an emulsion. Cracking can also occur if the oil turns rancid during storage. The acid formed denatures the emulsifying agent, causing the two phases to separate.

Cracking may occur due to addition of emulsifying agents of the opposite type or due to decomposition of the emulsifying agent

Creaming

It is the separation of the emulsion into two regions, one containing more of the disperse phase. In creaming, the oil separates out, forming a layer on top of the emulsion, but it usually remains in globules so that it can be redispersed on shaking (e.g. the cream on the top of boiled milk). This is undesirable as the product poor in appearance and if not shaken properly, there is a risk of the patient obtaining an incorrect dose. Creaming is less likely to occur if the viscosity of the continuous phase is increased.

Phase inversion

This is the process when an oil-in-water emulsion changes to a water-in-oil emulsion or from water-in-oil to oil-in-water emulsion. For stability of an emulsion, the optimum range of concentration of dispersed phase is 30–60% of the total volume. If the concentration of disperse phase exceeds this concentration, phase inversion occurs.

Auxiliary Label

SHAKE WELL BEFORE USE.

Liquid Paraffin Emulsion BP

Aim

To prepare and submit 20 ml Zinc Sulphide Lotion.

Synonym

Sulphurated Potash and Zinc lotion.

Sulphurated Potash lotion.

Formula

Sl. No	Ingredients	Official formula	Working formula
1	Sulphurated Potash	5 g	
2	Zinc Sulphate	5 g	
3	Concentrated Camphor water	2.5 ml	
4	Purified water (q.s)	100 ml	

Principle

Zinc Sulphide lotion is a suspension produced by chemical reaction. Here the insoluble active constituent (zinc sulphide) of the lotion is formed by a chemical reaction.

Sulphurated potash is a mixture of potassium polysulphides and other sulphur containing potassium compounds .It should be freshly prepared because the solubility of zinc sulphide decreases on storage.

Sulphurated potash reacts with Zinc sulphate to produce a precipitate of zinc sulphide that is diffusible in nature only if the sulphurated   potash is added to Zinc Sulphate.

If the Zinc Sulphate is added to sulphurated potash, then the precipitate formed will be indiffusible in nature.

A fine precipitate is obtained if dilute solutions of the reactants are mixed. Hence the reacting substances should be dissolved separately in approximately half the volume of the vehicle and the two parts mixed. If the suspension is prepared in this manner, the precipitate will be diffusible and no suspending agent is necessary.

Procedure

1. Sulphurated potash was dissolved in 50ml water.

2. Zinc Sulphate was also dissolved in 50 ml water.

3. Sulphurated potash solution was added slowly to the Zinc Sulphate solution with constant stirring.

4. Camphor water was added in small amounts with vigorous shaking to redissolve the precipitated camphor.

5. The suspension was made upto volume and mixed.

Category

Used in the treatment of acne and scabies.

Direction

To be applied on the skin with cotton.

Auxiliary label

SHAKE WELL BEFORE USE.

FOR EXTERNAL USE ONLY.

Storage

Store in a cool and dry place.

Cod Liver Oil Emulsion BP

Aim

To prepare and submit 20ml of cod liver oil emulsion.

Synonym

Emulsio Olei Morrhuae.

Formula

Sl. No	Ingredients	Official formula	Working formula
1	Cod liver oil	50 ml	
2	Acacia (powder)	12.5 g	
3	Tragacanth(powder)	0.7 g	
4	Saccharin Sodium	0.01 g	
5	Volatile bitter almond oil	0.1 ml	
6	Chloroform	0.2 ml	
7	Purified water (q.s)	100 ml	

Calculation of Primary Emulsion Formula

Since cod liver is a fixed oil, the formula for primary emulsion **is oil: water: gum** in the ratio **4:2:1**. Therefore the quantities for the primary emulsion are

Cod liver oil	-	50 ml
Water	-	25 ml
Acacia gum	-	12.5 g

Principle

This O/W emulsion is prepared by dry gum method using acacia gum as the primary emulsifying agent. Tragacanth is the secondary emulsifying agent and thickening agent. Bitter almond oil is the flavoring agent. Saccharin sodium is the sweetener. Chloroform acts as the preservative.

Procedure

1. The required quantities of gum acacia and tragacanth were taken into a mortar. The required quantity of cod liver oil was added and triturated rapidly to obtain a uniform mixture. The calculated quantity of purified water was added and triturated vigorously in a single direction till a clicking sound was produced and a thick creamy emulsion was formed.

   This is the PRIMARY EMULSION.

2. Saccharin sodium previously dissolved in a small quantity of purified water was added to the primary emulsion and triturated uniformly.

3. Bitter almond oil and chloroform were added and the emulsion was then made upto the volume with the remaining water.

Category

Source of Vitamin A and D.

Dosage

5ml daily for a 2-year-old child.

Auxiliary label

SHAKE WELL BEFORE USE.

Storage

Store in a cool and dry place.

Marketed Formulations

SEVENSEAS SEACOD COD LIVER OIL CAPSULES (Universal Medicare).

ELEVEN SEAS COD LIVER OIL CAPSULES (Taj Pharmaceuticals).

EXPERIMENT 36

Castor Oil Emulsion

Aim

To prepare and submit 20 ml of Castor oil emulsion.

Formula

Sl.No	Ingredients	Standard formula	Working formula
1	Castor oil	8 ml	
2	Acacia gum	2 g	
3	Purified water(q.s)	30 ml	

Calculation of Primary Emulsion Formula

Since castor oil is a fixed oil, the formula for primary emulsion is **oil: water: gum** in the ratio **4:2:1**. Therefore the quantities for the primary emulsion are

Castor oil	-	8 ml
Water	-	4 ml
Acacia gum	-	2 g

Principle

This emulsion is prepared by dry gum method using acacia gum as an emulsifying agent.

Procedure

1. The required quantity of castor oil was taken into a mortar. Calculated quantity of Gum acacia was added and triturated rapidly to obtain a uniform mixture. The calculated quantity of purified water was added and triturated vigorously in a single direction till a clicking sound was produced and a thick creamy emulsion was formed.

   This is the PRIMARY EMULSION.

2. The emulsion was then made upto volume with the remaining water.

Category

Mild irritant purgative.

Dosage

10ml to be taken in the morning before breakfast.

Auxiliary label

SHAKE WELL BEFORE USE.

Storage

Store in a cool and dry place.

EXPERIMENT 37

Liquid Paraffin and Magnesium Hydroxide Emulsion BPC

Aim

To prepare and submit 20 ml of Liquid Paraffin and Magnesium Hydroxide emulsion.

Synonym

Mixture of Magnesium hydroxide and Liquid Paraffin.

Emulsio Paraffini Liquidi et Magnesii Hydroxidi.

Formula

Sl. No	Ingredients	Official formula	Working formula
1	Liquid Paraffin	250 ml	
2	Magnesium hydroxide mixture	700 ml	
3	Chloroform spirit	50 ml	

Principle

This preparation is an internal emulsion emulsified with a finely divided solid. The emulgent is Magnesium Hydroxide mixture.

Finely divided solids with suitably balanced hydrophobic and hydrophilic properties are adsorbed at the oil- water interface forming a coherent film that prevents the coalescence of the dispersed globules. In this preparation, Chloroform spirit is the preservative.

Procedure

1. Chloroform spirit was mixed with Magnesium hydroxide mixture.

2. This mixture was then added to liquid paraffin in a bottle and shaken well.

3. The contents of the bottle were then passed through a hand homogenizer to obtain a stable emulsion.

Category

Laxative.

Dosage

5-20 ml

This preparation is best taken at bedtime preferably with water and if necessary, again in the morning or as advised by the physician.

Auxiliary label

SHAKE WELL BEFORE USE.

Storage

Store in a cool and dry place.

Marketed Formulations

CREMAFFIN (Abbott)

DUOLAXIN (Glenmark)

EXPERIMENT 38

Oily Calamine lotion BPC

Aim

To prepare and submit 20 ml of Oily Calamine lotion.

Synonym

Linimentum Calaminae.

Formula

Sl. No	Ingredients	Official formula	Working formula
1	Calamine	50 g	
2	Wool fat	10 g	
3	Arachis Oil	500 ml	
4	Oleic acid	5 ml	
5	Calcium Hydroxide Solution (q.s)	1000 ml	

Principle

Oily Calamine lotion is a 'Lime' cream type of lotion. They are W/O emulsions of fixed oils in which calcium soap is the emulsifying agent. In this lotion, 50% of Arachis oil is emulsified by lime soap produced from lime water and oleic acid. The emulsion is stabilized with wool fat.

Procedure

1. Wool fat, Arachis oil and Oleic acid were melted together.
2. Calamine was triturated with this molten mixture.
3. The creamy mass was then transferred to a suitable container; Calcium hydroxide solution was added to it and shaken vigorously.
4. The solution was then made up to volume with Calcium hydroxide solution and dispensed.

Category

Soothing application for the treatment of eczema.

Auxiliary label

FOR EXTERNAL USE ONLY.

SHAKE WELL BEFORE USE.

Storage

Store in a cool and dry place.

Calciferol Emulsion

Aim

To prepare and submit 20ml of Calciferol emulsion.

Formula

Sl. No	Ingredients	Standard formula	Working formula
1	Calciferol	3 ml	
2	Acacia (powder)	q.s	
3	Glycerin	6 ml	
4	Purified water (q.s)	100 ml	

The Percentage of calciferol in this preparation is 3 %. This should be increased to 20% by adding arachis oil.

Therefore the volume of arachis oil to be added is 20 ml – 3 ml = 17 ml for 100ml of the preparation.

Therefore the total quantity of oil will be: 3 ml of Calciferol together with 17 ml of Arachis oil.

Calculation of Primary Emulsion Formula

Since Calciferol is a fixed oil, the formula for primary emulsion **is oil: water: gum** in the ratio **4:2:1**. Therefore the quantities for the primary emulsion are

Calciferol   -   3 ml

Arachis oil   -   17 ml

Water	-	10 ml
Acacia gum	-	5 g

Principle

Acacia emulsions containing less than 20 % of oil cream readily. To prevent this a bland fixed oil such as arachis oil is added to increase the total oil content to approximately 20%.

In Calciferol emulsion, the concentration of Calciferol is 3%, therefore Arachis ioil is added to raise the oil content to 20%.

Procedure

1. The required quantities of gum acacia were taken into a mortar. The required quantity of Calciferol and Arachis oil were added and triturated rapidly to obtain a uniform mixture. The calculated quantity of purified water was added and triturated vigorously in a single direction till a clicking sound was produced and a thick creamy emulsion was formed.

   This is the PRIMARY EMULSION.

2. Glycerin was added to the primary emulsion and triturated uniformly.

3. Purified water was added to produce the required volume.

Category

Vitamin D supplement.

Dosage

As directed by the physician.

Auxiliary label

SHAKE WELL BEFORE USE.

Storage

Store in a cool and dry place.

Powders

Powders are intimate mixtures of dry, finely divided drugs and or chemicals that may be intended for internal administration or external application. They are available in crystalline or amorphous form.

Classification of Powders

1. Divided powders – Simple and compound powders for internal use.
2. Bulk powders for internal use.
3. Bulk powders for external use.
   - Dusting powders
   - Insufflations
   - Dentifrices
4. Effervescent powders.
5. Powders enclosed in cachets and capsules.

Advantages

1. They are more stable than liquid dosage forms.
2. Chances of incompatibility are less.
3. They can be consumed in bulk quantities along with food or by mixing in a suitable liquid.
4. They can easily be administered to children and elderly patients.
5. Since powders are in a fine state of sub division, they show faster dissolution and rapid onset of action, when compared to other solid dosage forms.
6. They are economical dosage forms since they do not require large machinery or special techniques of manufacture.
7. They are easy to carry than liquids.
8. They can be used internally as well as externally.

Disadvantages

1. Drugs having bitter, nauseous and unpleasant taste cannot be dispensed as powders.

2. Hygroscopic and deliquescent substances cannot be administered in powder form.

3. Drugs which are volatile in nature or prone to oxidation cannot be dispensed in powder form.

Eutectic Powder

Aim

To prepare and submit 3 packets of eutectic powder (Calculate 1 extra packet to account for any wastage).

Formula

Sl. No	Ingredients	Official formula (imperial system)	Official formula (metric system)	Working formula
1	Menthol	gr ii		
2	Camphor	gr iv		
3	Light magnesium carbonate	gr vi		

(The quantities mentioned are in imperial system and should be converted to metric system. The conversion factor is 1gr = 65mg /60mg)

Principle

When two organic substances having a low melting point are brought into physical contact with each other, they liquefy due to the formation of a new substance that has a melting point below room temperature. The reason for this change is that each ingredient acts as an impurity for the other, resulting in the lowering of the melting point of both the ingredients below room temperature and the mixture liquefies. Such substances are called "Eutectic substances".

E.g. Menthol, camphor, thymol, chloral hydrate, phenol, ammonium chloride, aspirin, phenyl salicylate etc.

Eutectic powders may be dispensed in two ways:

1. Dispense as separate set of powders, with directions that one set of each powder may be taken as a single dose.

2. They can also be dispensed by adding an inert substance such as kaolin, starch, lactose or light magnesium oxide. These substances act as absorbents and prevent liquefaction.

In this preparation light magnesium carbonate is the absorbent. Since camphor and menthol are volatile in nature, the powder has to be dispensed in double wrapped paper packets.

Procedure

1. Light magnesium carbonate was divided into two equal portions.

2. One portion was mixed with menthol and the other with camphor.

3. The two powder mixtures were then mixed together by spatulation.

4. The required quantity for each packet was weighed individually and double wrapped.

5. The powder packets were then tied with a paper band and dispensed in a neatly labeled white envelope.

Category

Anti- pruritic.

Auxiliary label

FOR EXTERNAL USE ONLY.

Storage

Store in a cool and dry place.

EXPERIMENT 41

Explosive Powder

Aim

To prepare and submit 4 packets of explosive powder (Calculate 1 extra packet to account for any wastage).

Formula

Sl. No	Ingredients	Standard formula	Batch formula	Working formula (for 1 extra pkt)
1	Potassium chlorate	0.6 g		
2	Tannic acid	0.3 g		
3	Sucrose	0.3 g		

Principle

When an oxidizing agent such as Potassium chlorate is triturated with a reducing agent such as tannic acid, it results in a violent explosion. Therefore each ingredient is triturated separately and mixed lightly with each other.

This preparation is used as a gargle. Potassium chlorate and tannic acid are astringents. Sucrose is used as diluent and sweetening agent.

Since tannic acid and sucrose are hygroscopic in nature, the powder has to be double wrapped.

E.g of other oxidizing agents are potassium dichromate, potassium nitrate, potassium permanganate, silver nitrate.

E.g of other reducing agents are charcoal, sulphur, sulphides.

Procedure

1. Sucrose was divided into 2 two parts.

2. The first part was triturated with potassium chlorate.

3. The second part was triturated with tannic acid.

4. Both the portions were mixed lightly and the required quantity for each packet was weighed individually and double wrapped.

5. The powder packets were then tied with a paper band and dispensed in a neatly labeled white envelope.

Category

Astringent

Direction

Dissolve one packet in a glass of water and use as a gargle.

Auxiliary label

NOT TO BE TAKEN ORALLY.

NOT TO BE SWALLOWED IN LARGE QUANTITIES.

Storage

Store in a cool and dry place.

Dusting Powder

Aim

To prepare and submit 10 g of dusting powder (Calculate 5g extra).

Formula

Sl. No	Ingredients	Standard formula	Batch formula	Working formula (for 5g extra)
1	Purified talc	50 g		
2	Starch powder	25 g		
3	Zinc oxide powder	25 g		

Principle

Dusting powders are preparations meant for external application to the intact or broken skin for their antiseptic, anti-pruritic, astringent, adsorbent, anti-perspirant and protective purposes. These powders must be homogenous and finely subdivided to enhance effectiveness and minimize local irritation. They should have good flowability, spreadability and should stick to the skin.

Dusting powders are of 2 types:

(a) **Medical dusting powder** – mainly used for superficial skin conditions. Sterility is rarely essential, but the powder must be free from dangerous pathogens. Medicated dusting powders are not intended for application to open wounds or broken skin.

(b) Surgical dusting powder – used in body cavities, on major wounds due to burns and on the umbilical cords of infants. They should be sterilized before use.

This preparation contains talc which is from mineral origin. The talc may be contaminated with spores of *Clostridium tetanii, Clostridium welchii* and *Bacillus anthracis*. Therefore it must be sterilized by heating at 160°C for 1 hour before use.

Dusting powders are dispensed in sifter top containers.

Procedure

1. All the ingredients were triturated to a fine powder separately and weighed.

2. The powders were then mixed in the ascending order of their weights.

3. The mixed powder was passed through sieve no 120 and mixed lightly.

4. The powder was then transferred to sifter top containers labeled and dispensed.

Category

Protective, antiseptic and absorbant.

Direction

Apply on the affected area twice or thrice a day.

Auxiliary label

FOR EXTERNAL USE ONLY.

NOT TO BE APPLIED ON CUT AND BROKEN SKIN.

Storage

Store in a cool and dry place.

Marketed Formulations

CANDID dusting powder (Glenmark Pharmaceuticals)

CLOBEN dusting powder (Indoco Remedies)

CLOCIP (Cipla)

EXPERIMENT 43

Insufflation

Aim

To prepare and submit 10 g of insufflation (Calculate 5g extra).

Formula

Sl. No	Ingredients	Standard formula	Batch formula	Working formula (for 5 g extra)
1	Ammonium chloride	30 g		
2	Menthol	5 g		
3	Camphor	5 g		
4	Light magnesium carbonate	60 g		

Principle

Insufflations are finely divided medicated powders meant for introduction into the body cavities such as ears, nose, throat, vagina and tooth sockets with the help of a device known as an insufflator.

In this preparation Ammonium chloride, menthol and camphor are eutectic substances. Therefore light magnesium carbonate is used as the absorbent to prevent liquefaction.

117

Procedure

1. Light magnesium carbonate was divided into three equal portions.
2. The first portion of magnesium carbonate was mixed with ammonium chloride, the second portion with menthol and the third portion with camphor.
3. The three powder mixtures were then mixed together by spatulation.
4. The powder mixture was then transferred to a suitable container.

Category

Expectorant.

Direction

To be used in a suitable atomizer as directed.

Auxiliary label

FOR EXTERNAL USE ONLY.

Storage

Store in a cool and dry place.

EXPERIMENT 44

Tooth Powder

Aim

To prepare and submit 10 g of Tooth Powder. (Calculate 5g extra).

Formula

Sl. No	Ingredients	Standard formula	Batch formula	Working formula (for 5 g extra)
1	Calcium Carbonate	92.8 g		
2	Soap powder	6 g		
3	Clove oil	1 ml		
4	Saccharin Sodium	0.2 g		

Principle

Tooth powders are preparations used to maintain oral hygiene. They are applied with the help of a toothbrush for cleaning the surface of the teeth and to remove the adhering layers without causing damage to the surface of the teeth.

In this preparation, calcium carbonate is used as the abrasive or cleaning and polishing agent.

Soap powder is the detergent. It provides foam to suspend and remove the debris.

Clove oil is the flavouring agent and also acts as a mild antiseptic. Sodium Saccharin is the sweetener. It is used in dentifrices, tooth pastes and other preparations for oral hygiene because it is less likely than carbohydrates to cause dental caries.

Procedure

1. Calcium Carbonate and Soap powder were triturated together.

2. Clove oil and saccharin Sodium were added and the trituration continued.

3. The triturated mixture was passed through sieve No. 120 to obtain a fine powder.

4. The powder mixture was then transferred to a sifter top container.

Category

Dentifrice.

Auxiliary label

FOR EXTERNAL USE ONLY.

Storage

Store in a cool and dry place.

EXPERIMENT 45

Face Powder

Aim

To prepare and submit 10 g of Face powder. (Calculate 5g extra).

Formula

Sl. No	Ingredients	Standard formula	Batch formula	Working formula (for 5g extra)
1	Kaolin	8 g		
2	Calcium Carbonate (light)	10 g		
3	Zinc Oxide	15 g		
4	Zinc Stearate	7 g		
5	Magnesium Carbonate	10 g		
6	Talc	50 g		
7	Perfume	q.s		

Principle

Face powders are cosmetic preparations used to impart a smooth finish to the skin and to mask minor visible imperfections and shine due to moisture or grease.

In the following preparation. Kaolin is used as an absorbent and to enhance the covering power (to mask minor imperfections on skin) of the powder.

Zinc Oxide is an antiseptic and mild astringent.

Zinc stearate and Talc are used to provide slip and adhesion properties to the powder. Slip is that quality of powder which makes it easy to spread and imparts a characteristic smooth feeling to the skin.

Magnesium carbonate is also an absorbent.

Procedure

1. All the ingredients were triturated to a fine powder separately and weighed.

2. The powders were then mixed in the ascending order of their weights.

3. The mixed powder was passed through sieve no 60 and mixed lightly.

4. The powder was then transferred to a suitable container.

Category

Cosmetic.

Direction

To be applied with a powder puff.

Auxiliary label

FOR EXTERNAL USE ONLY.

Storage

Store in a cool and dry place.

EXPERIMENT 46

Oral Rehydration Salts (ORS) IP

Aim

To prepare and submit 10 g of ORS powder (Calculate 5g extra).

Synonym

ORS Powder.

Formula

The composition of the formulation in terms of the amount in grams to be dissolved in sufficient water to produce 1000ml is given below.

Sl. No	Ingredients	Official formula	Working formula	Working formula (for 5 g extra)
1	Sodium Chloride	2.6 g		
2	Dextrose(anhydrous) Or Dextrose monohydrate	13.5 g 14.85 g		
3	Potassium Chloride	1.5 g		
4	Sodium Citrate	2.9 g		

Principle

Oral rehydration salts are dry, homogenously mixed powders containing Dextrose, Sodium chloride, Potassium Chloride and either Sodium Bicarbonate or Sodium Citrate. The mixture when mixed properly with clean water can help rehydrate the body when a lot of fluid has been lost.

Procedure

All ingredients were weighed and mixed in the increasing order of their weights.

Category

Replacement solution for diarrhoeal rehydration.

(i.e in the treatment and prevention of dehydration due to diarrrhoea and gastroenteritis in children and adults.

Direction

1. Add the contents of the ORS packet into a clean container. Add the correct amount of freshly boiled and cooled water. Stir well and feed it to the patient from a clean cup.

2. Any portion of the solution prepared from the oral powder that remains unused for 24 hrs after preparation should be discarded.

3. Do not add ORS to milk, soup, fruit juices or soft drinks.

Storage

Store in sachets made of aluminium foil. Store in a cool and dry place.

Marketed Formulations

ELECTRAL (FDC Spectra)

ORS-L (Juggat Pharma)

ELECTROKIND(Mankind Pharma)

ERO(Lupin)

EXPERIMENT 47

Compound Effervescent Powder BPC

Aim

To prepare and submit 2 packets of Compound effervescent powder.

Synonym

Seidlitz powder.

Pulvis Effervescens Compositus.

Formula

Sl.No	Ingredients	Official formula	Batch formula	Working formula (for 1 extra packet)
1.	Sodium Potassium Tartrate	7.5 g		
2.	Sodium Bicarbonate	2.5 g		
3.	Tartaric acid	2.5 g		

Principle

This preparation consists of 2 powders.

No.1 contains a mixture of Sodium Potassium Tartrate & Sodium Bicarbonate wrapped in blue paper.

No.2 contains tartaric acid wrapped in white paper.

Procedure

1. Sodium Potassium Tartrate & Sodium Bicarbonate were mixed and double wrapped.
2. Tartaric acid was double wrapped.
3. The packets were then dispensed in an envelope with proper labeling.

Category

Saline Purgative.

Direction

Add the contents of the blue and white packet to a glassful of cold or warm water and drink immediately.

Storage

Store in a cool and dry place. Both the packets should be stored separately.

Effervescent Granules

Aim

To prepare and submit 15 g of effervescent granules.

Formula

Sl.No	Ingredients	Standard formula	Batch formula	Working formula (for 5 g extra)
1	Citric acid	180g		
2	Tartaric acid	270g		
3	Sodium Bicarbonate	510g		
4	Sucrose	40g		

Principle

Effervescent granules contain a medicament mixed with citric acid, tartaric acid and sodium bicarbonate. A sweetening agent may be added. Before administration, they are dissolved in water; the acid and the bicarbonate react in the presence of water to produce effervescence, which is due to the release of carbon dioxide.

The carbonated water produced from the release of CO_2 serves to mask the bitter and saline taste of drugs. It also stimulates the flow of gastric juice and helps in the absorption of the medicament. The quantity of acids used is slightly more than the quantity actually required for complete neutralization of Sodium bicarbonate because the preparations with a slightly acidic taste are more palatable.

Citric acid contains one molecule of water of crystallization, which is liberated during heating and serves as the moistening agent for the powders during granulation. If citric acid is used alone, it will liberate its water of crystallization during heating, thus making the mass too wet for sieving.

$$3\ NaHCO_3\ +\ C_6H_8O_7.H_2O\ \longrightarrow\ C_6H_5Na_3O_7\ +\ 3CO_2\uparrow\ +\ 4H_2O$$

$$\text{Citric acid} \qquad\qquad \text{Sodium citrate}$$

If tartaric acid is used alone, it is anhydrous and another solvent will have to be used for granule preparation and the resulting granules will lose their firmness and readily crumble. Citric acid partially neutralizes sodium bicarbonate and the rest is neutralized by tartaric acid.

$$2\ NaHCO_3\ +\ C_4H_6O_6\ \longrightarrow\ C_4H_4Na_2O_6\ +\ 2\ CO_2\uparrow\ +\ 2H_2O$$

$$\text{Tartaric acid} \qquad\qquad \text{Sodium Tartrate}$$

Therefore citric acid and tartaric acid is used in combination.

In the following preparation, sucrose is used as the sweetening agent. Before administration, the granules should be dissolved in water and consumed immediately.

Procedure

1. All the ingredients were triturated to a fine powder, weighed and transferred to a preheated china dish.

2. The citric acid looses its water of crystallization and makes the powder mixture moist.

3. When the powder mixture became a damp mass, it was passed through sieve no 6 to obtain granules.

4. The granules were then dried at a temperature not exceeding 54°C, passed through sieve no. 20 and filled into airtight containers.

Category

Saline purgative.

Direction

Dissolve one teaspoonful in a glass of water and consume immediately.

Auxiliary label

REPLACE THE CAP IMMEDIATELY AFTER USE.

Storage

Store in an airtight container in a cool and dry place.

Suppositories

Suppositories are solid unit dosage forms suitably shaped for insertion into the rectum. The bases used either melt when warmed to body temperature or dissolve or disperse when in contact with mucous secretions. Suppositories may contain medicaments, dissolved or dispersed in the base, which are intended to exert a systemic or a local effect.

Advantages

1. Suppositories are employed to provide a local effect for the treatment of infection and inflammation, e.g. haemorrhoids. Rectal dosage forms are used to promote evacuation of the bowel (by irritating the rectum), to relieve constipation or to cleanse the bowel prior to surgery.

2. Suppositories may be employed to provide systemic drug absorption in situations where oral drug absorption is not recommended, in cases such as:

   - Patients who are unconscious, e.g. patients in intensive care or in postoperative patients.

   - Patients who are vomiting, e.g. gastrointestinal infection, migraine.

   - Gastro irritant drugs, e.g. non-steroidal anti-inflammatory agents, particularly in chronic usage.

   - Drugs that undergo degradation in the stomach.

   - Drugs that are erratically absorbed from the upper gastrointestinal tract.

   - Administration of the drugs that undergo extensive first-pass metabolism. If administered correctly, the therapeutic agent is absorbed directly into the systemic circulation, thereby avoiding direct entry into the liver.

3. Rectal dosage forms may be employed to provide local treatment of diseases of the colon, e.g. Crohn's disease, ulcerative colitis.

Disadvantages

1. May be unacceptable to certain patients.
2. May be difficult to self administer by arthritic or physically compromised patients.
3. Unpredictable and variable absorption *in vivo*.

Suppository Bases

The ideal properties of a suppository base include:

1. The base should be solid at the storage temperature of the formulation but should soften, melt or dissolve in the rectal fluid following insertion into the rectum, thereby releasing the drug.
2. The base should retain its shape during handling.
3. The base should be non toxic and non-irritant to the rectal mucosa.
4. The base should be compatible with the other ingredients.
5. The base should be chemically and physically stable over the period of storage (shelf-life).
6. The base should be easily moulded and should not adhere to the mould.

The types of suppository base are:

(a) Fatty or oleaginous bases - melt at body temperature.
   - Cocoa butter (Theobroma oil)
   - Emulsified theobroma oil
   - Hydrogenated oils

(b) Water soluble or water miscible bases- dissolve or disperse in the rectal secretions.
   - Glycerol- gelatin base
   - Soap glycerin bases
   - Macrogols

(c) Emulsifying bases.
   - Witepsol
   - Massa Estarinum
   - Massuppol

Fatty (oleaginous) Bases

Fatty bases are predominantly composed of naturally occurring or semi synthetic/synthetic fatty acid esters of glycerol. These bases melt quickly at body temperature.

Cocoa Butter (theobroma oil)

It is a yellowish white solid obtained from the crushed and roasted seeds of Theobroma cocoa. Mainly consists of a mixture of glyceryl esters of stearic, palmitic, oleic and other fatty acids. The presence of unsaturated (e.g. oleic acid) esters contributes to the low melting point of cocoa butter (30–36^0C), thereby facilitating rapid melting on insertion into the rectum.

The major disadvantages of cocoa butter as a suppository base are:

1. *Polymorphism:* which is the ability of this material to exist in different crystalline forms.

   If cocoa butter is melted at 36^0C and allowed to solidify slowly, the stable β (beta) polymorph will form. The β crystals melts between 34 and 36^0C But if over heated, it may produce on cooling, unstable γ (gamma) crystals which melt at 15^0C or α (alpha) crystals which melt at $20°C$. These unstable forms return to the stable conditions after several days.

   The melting/softening point of cocoa butter may be too low for storage at room temperature and therefore either storage under controlled temperature or the inclusion of excipients that raise the melting/softening temperature of cocoa butter (e.g. beeswax, cetyl esters wax) may be required.

2. *Adherence to the mould:* Since theobroma oil doesn't contract enough on cooling to loosen the suppositories in the mould, sticking will occur. To prevent this, the mould should be lubricated before use.

3. *Softening point is too low for hot climates:* To overcome this problem, beeswax (4- 5% w/w) or cetyl esters wax (20% w/w) may be added to the suppository to raise the softening point.

4. **Melting point is reduced by soluble ingredients:** Substances such as chloral hydrate that dissolve in theobroma oil may lower its melting point to such an extent that the suppositories become too soft to use. To restore the melting point, a controlled amount of white bees wax (4-5%) may be added. If more is used, the suppository may not melt at room temperature.

5. ***Slow deterioration during storage:*** which is due to the oxidation of unsaturated glycerides.

6. ***Poor water absorbing capacity:*** can be improved by the addition of an emulsifying agent.

7. ***Leakage from the body:*** Sometimes the melted base escapes from the rectum or vagina. This may happen with pessaries and therefore are rarely made with theobroma oil.

Water-Soluble and Water-Miscible Bases

These bases do not melt at body temperature but dissolves in the body fluids.

Glycerol-Gelatin

This suppository base is prepared by dissolving gelatin (20% w/w) in glycerol (70% w/w) with the aid of heating (100^0C). The required drug is generally dissolved/dispersed in an aqueous phase (< 10% w/w) and then combined with the glycerol phase with stirring prior to pouring into the suppository mould.

Glycerol–gelatin bases may be used for the formulation of suppositories that contain a water-soluble therapeutic agent. The use of base is restricted by several disadvantages, like:

1. An associated physiological effect- E.g. laxative action and can be used for this purpose to relieve constipation or to facilitate bowel evacuation prior to surgery.

2. Difficult to prepare and handle.

3. Hygroscopic- Glycerol–gelatin bases will absorb moisture from the atmosphere and therefore must be carefully packaged to prevent entry of moisture. This ability of glycerol–gelatin bases to absorb water will also occur within the rectum, leading to dehydration and irritation of the rectal mucosa. This action prompts bowel evacuation. To minimize this, the suppository may be moistened with water prior to insertion.

4. Potential interactions with therapeutic agents- gelatin is incompatible with tannic acid, ferric chloride etc.

Macrogols

Water-miscible bases are composed of PEGs possessing a molecular weight greater than 1000 g/mol. The melting point of these higher grades of PEGs increases as the molecular weight increases, e.g. the melting points of PEG 1000 and PEG 8000 are 37–40^{0}C and 60–63^{0}C, respectively.

Following insertion into the rectum, these suppositories will not melt but dissolve gradually to release the drug.

The disadvantages of this base are:

1. These bases are hygroscopic in nature and can cause discomfort to the patient due to the extraction of water from the rectal mucosa into the suppository. This may be minimized by the inclusion of water (> 20% w/w) or by moistening the suppository prior to insertion.

2. Since PEG-based suppositories are hygroscopic in nature, they have to be stored in moisture-resistant packaging.

3. PEG also enhances the solubility of therapeutic agents and therefore this interaction between the drug and polymer will prevent the release of the drug from the liquefied base, resulting in decreased therapeutic activity.

4. The high solubility of the drug in the solid base may change with storage conditions and time resulting in crystal growth within the suppository. Crystal growth can fracture the product on storage.

Formulation of Suppositories

The other excipients present in suppository formulations include:

1. *Surface-active agents:* These are included to enhance the wetting properties of the suppository base with the rectal fluid. This in turn will enhance drug release/dissolution. The use of surfactants is mainly reserved for formulations composed of a lipophilic suppository base and/or a lipophilic drug. E.g. sorbitan esters (Spans) and polyoxyethylene sorbitan fatty acid esters (Tweens).

2. *Agents to reduce hygroscopicity:* e.g. colloidal silicon dioxide, may be included in fatty suppository bases to reduce the uptake of water from the atmosphere during storage and, in so doing, the physical and chemical stability of the dosage form may be enhanced.

3. *Agents to control the melting point of the base:* Substances such as phenol and chloral hydrate have a tendency to lower the melting point of cocoa butter. To overcome this problem, solidifying agents

like beeswax (4%) or cetyl esters wax (about 20%) may be melted with the cocoa butter.

The melting point of PEG-based suppositories may also be controlled by including higher molecular weight PEG's and the melting point of water-miscible suppository bases may be lowered by incorporating the required concentration of low-molecular-weight PEG (PEG 400).

Preparation of Suppositories

Suppositories are manufactured by moulding method. The base is heated to above the melting temperature, the drug dispersed (or dissolved) in the heated liquid and the molten mass is poured into suppository moulds. This is then allowed to cool, removed and packed.

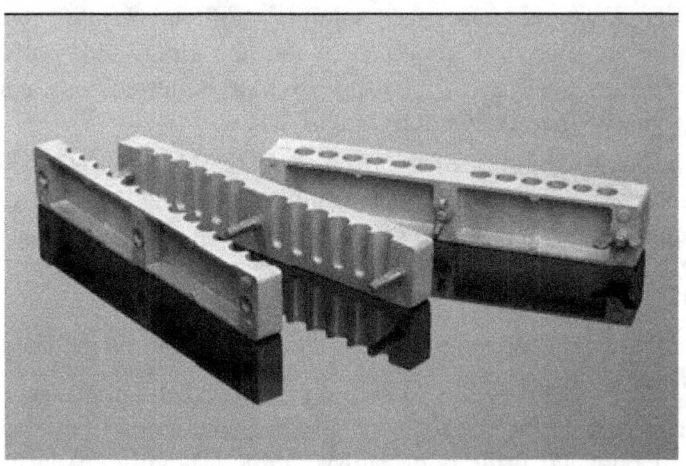

Suppository mould used in the manufacture of suppositories.

Lubrication of Moulds

Suppositories prepared using cocoa butter is prone to sticking in the metallic suppository mould after cooling. To prevent this, the moulds are usually lubricated before the molten mixture is poured to facilitate clean and easy removal of the moulded suppositories. Lubrication is not necessary for emulsifying bases or macrogols as they contract sufficiently on cooling, allowing easy removal.

The composition of the lubricant must differ from that of the base to prevent any interaction.

i.e. if the base is fatty, the lubricant must be aqueous and if the base is water soluble, the lubricant must be fatty in nature.

E.g. For cocoa butter suppositories: the lubricating solution is a mixture of soft soap, glycerin and 90% alcohol.

The lubricant should be applied with the help of a brush or a swab made of gauze. Cotton wool should not be used as it can leave behind the fibres on the mould.

Calibration of Moulds

Each individual mould is capable of holding a specific volume of material in each of its cavities. Because of the difference in the densities of the materials, the weight of the suppositories will vary with different bases. Similarly any added medicinal agent will alter the density of the base and the weight of the resulting suppositories will be different from that of those prepared with the base alone. Therefore each suppository mould should be calibrated before use.

Displacement Value

The volume of a suppository from a particular mould is same, but the weight varies. This is because the densities of the medicaments will vary from the density of the base. To obtain a product of uniform and accurate weight, allowance must be made for the change in density of the mass due to the added drugs. For this purpose displacement value is calculated.

"Displacement value is defined as the number of parts by weight of the medicament that displaces one part by weight of the base."

The displacement values for some of the medicaments with cocoa butter as the base are -

Aminophylline	1.5
Aspirin	1.3
Boric acid	1.5
Castor oil	1.0
Chloral hydrate	1.5
Tannic acid	1.0
Zinc oxide	5.0

Auxiliary Label

FOR RECTAL USE ONLY (in case of Suppositories)

FOR VAGINAL USE ONLY (in case of Pessaries)

Marketed Formulations

JUSTINSUPP (Neon Laboratories)

GYNASAFE PESSARIES (Taj pharmaceuticals)

TODAY PESSARIES (Bliss)

WOKADINE VAG (Wockhardt)

CANDID-CL (Glenmark)

EXPERIMENT 49

Boric Acid Suppositories

Aim

To prepare and submit 6 Boric acid suppositories (Calculate for 8).

Formula

Sl.No	Ingredients	Standard formula	Working formula
1.	Boric acid	120 mg	
2.	Cocoa butter (q.s)	1 g	

(Displacement value of boric acid is 1.5)

Formula for mould lubricant

Soft soap	10 g
Glycerin	10 g
Alcohol (90%)	50 ml

Calculations

1. Weight of boric acid for 1 suppository   =   120 mg

   Weight of boric acid for 8 suppositories   =   960 mg = 0.96 g

2. Weight of cocoa butter for 1 suppository   =   1 g

   Weight of cocoa butter for 8 suppositories =   8 g

Displacement value of boric acid is 1.5

i.e., 1.5 g of boric acid displaces 1 g of cocoa butter.

Therefore 0.96g of boric acid displaces = 0.96 / 1.5 = 0.64 g of cocoa butter.

Therefore the total weight of cocoa butter required = 8 g – 0.64 g = 7.36 g.

Principle

In the following preparation, boric acid is used as an antiseptic. Cocoa butter is a fatty base, which melts at body temperature, releasing the drug.

Suppositories are prepared in moulds. Lubricating the moulds allows easy removal of the suppositories. The cold mould is used for dissipating the heat content of the suppository mass and hastening setting. The mould is overfilled with molten drug + base mixture. This is because while cooling the base contracts forming a hollow cavity at the center top of the suppositories. Overfilling the mould prevents the formation of the cavity.

Each mould can be used to prepare six suppositories, but calculations are done for two extra suppositories (6 + 2) in order to compensate for the loss that occurs during preparation.

Procedure

1. The inner surface of the suppository mould was cleaned gently with luke warm detergent solution and rinsed with purified water.

2. The inner surfaces of the mould was lubricated by applying a thin smear of prepared mould lubricant and kept inverted on ice bath to drain the excess lubricant.

3. The calculated quantity of cocoa butter was heated in a china dish. When 3/4th of the base has melted, the dish was removed from the water bath and the mixture was stirred well until the remaining base also melts.

4. The weighed quantity of boric acid was placed on an ointment tile. Half of the molten base was poured over it and mixed thoroughly.

5. The mixed mass was again transferred to the china dish and warmed for a few seconds until it became pourable.

6. The molten mixture was then poured into the lubricated moulds until it overflows.

7. The mould was allowed to cool on an ice bath for 20-30 minutes. The excess of the mass was then scraped off with a sharp knife.

8. The mould was later unscrewed to remove the solidified suppositories.

9. Each suppository was wrapped in aluminium foils and dispensed.

Category

Antiseptic and local anti- infective.

Direction

- Insert one at night.

- Rub the suppositories gently with the fingers to melt the surface to provide lubrication for insertion.

Auxiliary label

FOR RECTAL USE ONLY.

Storage

Store in a cool and dry place.

Chloral Hydrate Suppositories

Aim

To prepare and submit 6 chloral hydrate suppositories (Calculate for 8).

Formula

Sl.No	Ingredients	Standard formula	Working formula
1	Chloral hydrate	60 mg	
2	Cocoa butter (q.s)	1 g	

(Displacement value of chloral hydrate is 1.5)

Formula for mould lubricant

Soft soap	10 g
Glycerin	10 g
Alcohol (90%)	50 ml

Calculations

1. Weight of chloral hydrate for 1 suppository =   60 mg

   Weight of chloral hydrate for 8 suppositories = 480 mg = 0.48 g

2. Weight of cocoa butter for 1 suppository = 1 g

Weight of cocoa butter for 8 suppositories = 8 g

Displacement value of chloral hydrate is 1.5

i.e. 1.5 g of chloral hydrate displaces 1 g of cocoa butter.

Therefore 0.48g of chloral hydrate displaces = 0.48 / 1.5 = 0.32 g of cocoa butter.

Therefore the total weight of cocoa butter required = 8 g – 0.32 g = 7.68 g.

Principle

In the following preparation, Chloral hydrate is used a sedative and hypnotic. Cocoa butter is a fatty base, which melts at body temperature, releasing the drug.

Substances such as chloral hydrate that dissolve in cocoa butter may lower its melting point to such an extent that the suppositories are too soft for use. To restore the melting point, a controlled amount of white bees wax (4-5 %) may be added. If more amount of beeswax is added, the suppositories may not melt at body temperature.

Procedure

1. The inner surface of the suppository mould was cleaned gently with luke warm detergent solution and rinsed with purified water.

2. The inner surfaces of the mould was lubricated by applying a thin smear of prepared mould lubricant and kept inverted on ice bath to drain the excess lubricant.

3. The calculated quantity of cocoa butter was heated in a china dish. When 3/4th of the base has melted, the dish was removed from the water bath and the mixture was stirred well until the remaining base also melts.

4. The weighed quantity of Chloral hydrate was placed on an ointment tile. Half of the molten base was poured over it and mixed thoroughly.

5. The mixed mass was again transferred to the china dish and warmed for a few seconds until it became pourable.

6. The molten mixture was then poured into the lubricated moulds until it overflows.

7. The mould was allowed to cool on an ice bath.

8. The excess of the mass was then scraped off with a sharp knife. The mould was later unscrewed to remove the solidified suppositories.

9. Each suppository was wrapped in aluminium foils and dispensed.

Category

Sedative and Hypnotic.

Direction

- Insert one at night.

- Rub the suppositories gently with the fingers to melt the surface to provide lubrication for insertion.

Auxiliary label

FOR RECTAL USE ONLY.

Storage

Store in a cool and dry place.

Zinc Oxide Suppositories

Aim

To prepare and submit 6 Zinc oxide suppositories (Calculate for 8).

Formula

Sl.No	Ingredients	Standard formula	Working formula
1	Zinc Oxide	400 mg	
2	Cocoa butter (q.s)	1 g	

(Displacement value of zinc oxide is 5.0)

Formula for mould lubricant

Soft soap	10 g
Glycerin	10 g
Alcohol (90%)	50 ml

Calculations

1. Weight of Zinc oxide for 1 suppository = 400 mg

   Weight of Zinc oxides for 8 suppositories = 3200 mg = 3.2 g

2. Weight of cocoa butter for 1 suppository = 1 g

   Weight of cocoa butter for 8 suppositories = 8 g

Displacement value of zinc oxide is 5.0

i.e., 5.0 g of zinc oxide displaces 1 g of cocoa butter.

Therefore 3.2 g of zinc oxide displaces = 3.2 / 5 = 0.64 g of cocoa butter.

Therefore the total weight of cocoa butter required = 8 g – 0.64 g = 7.36 g.

Principle

In the following preparation, Zinc oxide is used as an antiseptic. Cocoa butter is a fatty base, which melts at body temperature, releasing the drug. Suppositories are prepared in moulds. Lubricating the moulds allows easy removal of the suppositories. The cold mould is used for dissipating the heat content of the suppository mass and hastening setting. The mould is overfilled with molten drug + base mixture. This is because while cooling the base contracts forming a hollow cavity at the center top of the suppositories. Overfilling the mould prevents the formation of the cavity.

Each mould can be used to prepare six suppositories, but calculations are done for two extra suppositories (6 + 2) in order to compensate for the loss that occurs during preparation.

Procedure

1. The inner surface of the suppository mould was cleaned gently with luke warm detergent solution and rinsed with purified water.

2. The inner surfaces of the mould was lubricated by applying a thin smear of prepared mould lubricant and kept inverted on ice bath to drain the excess lubricant.

3. The calculated quantity of cocoa butter was heated in a china dish. When 3/4th of the base has melted, the dish was removed from the water bath and the mixture was stirred well until the remaining base also melts.

4. The weighed quantity of zinc oxide was placed on an ointment tile. Half of the molten base was poured over it and mixed thoroughly.

5. The mixed mass was again transferred to the china dish and warmed for a few seconds until it became pourable.

6. The molten mixture was then poured into the lubricated moulds until it overflows.

7. The mould was allowed to cool on an ice bath for 20-30 minutes. The excess of the mass was then scraped off with a sharp knife.

8. The mould was later unscrewed to remove the solidified suppositories.

9. Each suppository was wrapped in aluminium foils and dispensed.

Category

Antiseptic.

Direction

- Insert one at night.

- Rub the suppositories gently with the fingers to melt the surface to provide lubrication for insertion.

Auxiliary label

FOR RECTAL USE ONLY.

Storage

Store in a cool and dry place.

Glycerol Suppositories BP

Aim

To prepare and submit 6 Glycerol suppositories BP (Calculate for 8).

Formula

Sl.No	Ingredients	Standard formula	Working formula
1	Glycerol	70 g	
2	Gelatin	20 g	
3	Purified water (q.s)	100 g	

Calculations

There are 3 sizes of glycerol suppositories.

Size	Mould size (g)	Intended for
Small	1	Infants
Medium	2	Children
Large	4	Adults

The quantity of mass for 8 suppositories is $8 \times 4 \times 1.2 = 38.4$ g

Where

8 is the total number of suppositories to be prepared.

4 is the size of the mould (meant for adult use).

1.2 is the density factor.

Principle

Glycerol suppositories are made with Glycero-gelatin base. This base is a mixture of glycerol (70%w/w) and water made into a stiff jelly by adding gelatin (14%w/w). Glycero-gelatin base is water soluble in nature and dissolves in body secretions. Glycero-gelatin bases may be used unmedicated or medicated. These bases have a tendency to absorb moisture as a result of the hygroscopic nature of glycerine and must be protected from atmospheric moisture if they are to maintain their shape and consistency. Also as a result of the hygroscopicity of the glycerin, the suppository may have a dehydrating effect and irritate the tissues upon insertion. The water in the formula for the suppositories minimizes this action; however, if necessary, the suppositories may be moistened with water prior to insertion to reduce the initial tendency of the base to draw water from the mucous membranes and irritate the tissues.

The mass of Glycerol suppositories is 1.2 times as dense as theobroma oil and this is taken into account while calculating the required weight of base. Hence, when appropriate, displacement values are used in the normal way and after the amount of base has been calculated it is multiplied by the density factor 1.2.

Because the base is highly sticky, manipulation losses are high and quantities for 10 should be prepared when six 1 or 2 g suppositories need to be dispensed. If 4g products are required, calculations can be done for 2 extra suppositories. Each mould can be used to prepare six suppositories, but calculations are done for two extra suppositories (8 + 2) in order to compensate for the loss that occurs during preparation.

Suppositories are prepared in moulds. Lubricating agent used is liquid paraffin or arachis oil. The cold mould is used for dissipating the heat content of the suppository mass and hastening setting. Overfilling of the mould is not necessary because Glycero-gelatin bases contract very little on cooling and also because the excess mass cannot be neatly removed.

Procedure

1. The inner surface of the suppository mould was cleaned gently with luke warm detergent solution and rinsed with purified water.

2. The inner surfaces of the mould was lubricated by applying a thin smear of liquid paraffin or arachis oil and kept inverted on ice bath to drain the excess lubricant.

3.   The calculated quantity of glycerol was heated in a china dish to 100^0C and kept hot on a water bath.

4.   Weighed quantity of powdered gelatin was added to a small quantity of water and stirred gently to completely wet it.

5.   To the moistened gelatin, hot glycerol was added and stirred.

6.   The mixture was again transferred to a boiling water bath and heated until complete solubilization.

7.   When solution was completed, the contents were weighed and if necessary, evaporated or hot purified water was added to obtain the required weight.

8.   The hot mass was then poured into the lubricated moulds.

9.   The mould was allowed to cool on an ice bath for 20-30 minutes.

10.   The mould was later unscrewed to remove the solidified suppositories.

11.   Each suppository was made to stand on its base on a tile, previously lubricated with liquid paraffin or oil. The base was carefully trimmed with a sharp blade and the suppository was rolled on each tile to provide a slight coating o lubricant.

12.   Each suppository was wrapped in aluminium foils and dispensed.

Category

Laxative.

Direction

As directed by the physician.

Auxiliary label

FOR RECTAL USE ONLY.

Storage

Store in a airtight packages in a cool and dry place.

Collodions

Collodions are liquid preparations for external use. They are non-aqueous solutions of Pyroxylin in ether-alcohol with or without medicaments. They are meant for application to the skin and eave behind a film on drying.

The volatile solvents are ether and alcohol. The film producing ingredient is Pyroxylin (nitrocellulose) and the substance giving flexibility is castor oil.

Pyroxylin is obtained by the action of a mixture of nitric acid and sulphuric acid on defatted cotton.

Unmedicated collodions are useful for protecting small cuts and abrasions. Medicated collodions provide prolonged contact between the skin and a medicament.

The addition of 2% camphor and 3% castor oil to collodion renders the product flexible, permitting its comfortable use over skin areas that are normally moved such as fingers and toes.

Collodions should be applied with a fine camel hair brush or glass rod. On application, the solvent rapidly evaporates leaving a protective film of pyroxylin on the skin. This provides an occlusive protective coating to the skin.

Auxiliary Label

For external use only.

Highly inflammable.

Keep away from naked flame.

EXPERIMENT 53

Salicylic Acid Collodion BP

Aim

To prepare and submit 20ml of Salicylic Acid Collodion.

Synonym

Corn solvent.

Formula

Sl.No	Ingredients	Standard formula	Working formula
1	Salicylic acid	100 g	
2	Flexible Collodion (q.s)	1000 ml	

Preparation of Flexible Collodion

Pyroxylin	16 g
Colophony	30 g
Castor oil	30 g
Camphor	20 g
Alcohol (90%)	240 ml
Solvent ether (q.s)	1000 ml

Principle

Salicylic acid collodion is used for its keratolytic effects in the removal of corns from toes. Salicylic acid collodion is a 10% solution of salicylic

153

acid in flexible collodion. Pyroxylin (cellulose nitrate) is the film former. Colophony is added to improve adhesion and camphor makes the product waterproof. Castor oil is used as the plasticizer to make the collodion flexible. Solvent ether is the solvent.

Special care is essential while using this preparation. The product should be applied one drop at a time onto the wart or corn, allowing time to dry before the next drop is applied. As salicylic acid is irritating to normal and healthy skin, every attempt must be made to ensure application directly onto the corn or wart. The useful preventive measure is to line the adjacent healthy skin with some white petroleum jelly prior to the application of the product.

The vehicle is volatile and should be stored in well-closed containers.

Procedure

1. Pyroxylin was immersed in Alcohol (90%).

2. Colophony, camphor and castor oil were added to it.

3. Sufficient ether was added to produce 1000 ml.

4. The preparation is shaken well and set aside. The clear liquid was then decanted and used as Flexible collodion.

5. The required amount of Salicylic acid was weighed, mixed with flexible collodion in a container and shaken well until a uniform mixture was formed.

Category

Keratolytic (Corn solvent).

Direction

Apply with a brush one drop at a time on the corn or wart. Allow to dry before the next drop is applied.

Auxiliary label

FOR EXTERNAL USE ONLY.

HIGHLY INFLAMMABLE.

KEEP AWAY FROM NAKED FLAME.

Storage

Store in a well-closed container in a cool and dry place.

Lotions

Lotions are liquid preparations intended for application to the skin. The inclusion of alcohol in a lotion hastens its drying and imparts a cooling effect to the skin. The inclusion of glycerol keeps the skin moist for a long time.

Lotions are applied, without friction, on a soft absorbent fabric and covered with a waterproof material or dabbed on the skin.

Auxiliary Label

FOR EXTERNAL USE ONLY.

Containers

Lotion are supplied in coloured fluted bottles or in suitable plastic containers.

EXPERIMENT 54

Salicylic Acid Lotion BPC

Aim

To prepare and submit 20 ml of Salicylic acid lotion.

Synonym

Lotio Acidi Salicylici.

Formula

Sl. No	Ingredients	Official formula	Working formula
1	Salicylic Acid	20 g	
2	Castor Oil	10 ml	
3	Alcohol (95%) (q.s)	1000 ml	

Principle

Salicylic acid lotion is meant for external application to the skin with the help of an absorbent material. It is used for its antiseptic and astringent properties. Salicylic acid lotion can also be used as a fungicidal in dandruff treatment.

Alcohol provides cooling and soothing effect when the lotion is applied to the skin. Since alcohol is added in high concentrations, the defatting action is countered by the addition of castor oil.

Since the preparation contains large concentration of alcohol, it is highly inflammable. If the preparation is to be used for scalp conditions, then the container should be labeled as "This preparation is inflammable. Do not use it or dry the hair near a fire or naked flame".

Procedure

1. Salicylic acid was dissolved in a small portion of alcohol.

2. Castor oil was added to it.

3. Sufficient alcohol was added to produce the required volume and mixed well.

Category

Antiseptic and Astringent.

Auxiliary label

FOR EXTERNAL USE ONLY.

SHAKE WELL BEFORE USE.

THIS PREPARATION IS INFLAMMABLE. DO NOT USE IT NEAR A FIRE OR NAKED FLAME.

Storage

Store in a well-closed container in a cool and dry place.

Aminobenzoic Acid Lotion BPC

Aim

To prepare and submit 20 ml of Aminobenzoic Acid Lotion.

Formula

Sl. No	Ingredients	Official formula	Working formula
1	Aminobenzoic acid	50 g	
2	Glycerol	200 ml	
3	Alcohol (95%)	600 ml	
4	Purified water (q.s)	1000 ml	

Principle

Aminobenzoic acid has sun screening properties and is used as an ingredient of topical preparations for the prevention of sunburn.

Alcohol provides a cooling effect when the preparation is applied on the skin. Alcohol also enhances the solubility of Aminobenzoic acid. Glycerol is a humectant and keeps the skin moist.

Procedure

1. Aminobenzoic acid was dissolved in alcohol.
2. Glycerol was added to the solution and mixed well.
3. Purified water was added to produce the required volume.

Category

Sunscreen (used in the prevention of sunburn).

Auxiliary label

FOR EXTERNAL USE ONLY.

THE LOTION MAY STAIN CLOTHING.

Storage

Store in a cool and dry place. Protect from light.

Mouthwashes and Gargles

Mouthwashes are liquid preparations used to cleanse and deodorize the buccal cavity. They have a pleasant taste and odour and are very refreshing in nature. They are used to maintain oral hygiene.

Direction for Usage

Dilute with warm water before use.

Auxiliary Label

FOR EXTERNAL USE ONLY.

NOT TO BE TAKEN.

NOT TO BE SWALLOWED IN LARGE AMOUNTS.

Containers

Mouthwashes are dispensed in clear, fluted bottles.

Marketed Formulations

LISTERINE MOUTHWASH (Pfizer)

COLGATE PLAX MOUTHWASH

CHLORHEXIDINE MOUTHWASH (AHPL)

ORAL – B SENSITIVE

A.M-P.M MOUTHWASH (Elder Pharmaceuticals)

TANTUM ORAL RINSE(Elder Pharmaceuticals)

Gargles are aqueous solutions used to relieve soreness in mild throat infections. They are brought into close contact with the mucous membranes of the throat, allowed to remain there for a few seconds and then thrown out of the mouth.

Gargles are dispensed in concentrated form with directions to dilute with warm water before use.

Direction for Usage

Dilute with warm water before use.

Auxiliary Label

FOR EXTERNAL USE ONLY.

NOT TO BE TAKEN.

NOT TO BE SWALLOWED IN LARGE AMOUNTS.

Containers

Gargles are dispensed in clear, fluted glass bottles with a plastic screw cap.

Marketed Formulations

BETADINE GARGLE (Win- Medicare Pharmaceuticals)

IODOLAN GARGLE (East India)

EXPERIMENT 56

Compound Sodium Chloride Mouthwash BP

Aim

To prepare and submit 20 ml of Compound Sodium chloride mouthwash.

Synonym

Collutorium Sodii Chloridi Compositum.

Formula

Sl.No	Ingredients	Official formula	Working formula
1	Sodium chloride	15 g	
2	Sodium bicarbonate	10 g	
3	Concentrated Peppermint water (q.s)	25 ml	
4	Double strength chloroform water	500 ml	
5	Purified water (q.s)	1000 ml	

Principle

Mouthwashes are medicated liquids, which are used to clean and deodorize the buccal cavity. They are pleasant in taste and odour. They are formulated either in ready to use form or as concentrated

163

preparations. If they are dispensed in concentrated form, they are required to be diluted before use.

Procedure

1. Sodium chloride and Sodium bicarbonate were dissolved in a small quantity of peppermint water.
2. The solution was then made up to volume with the remaining peppermint water.

Category

Used to clean and freshen the mouth.

Direction

Use approximately 15 ml diluted with an equal volume of water every morning and night.

Auxiliary label

FOR EXTERNAL USE ONLY.

NOT TO BE TAKEN.

NOT TO BE SWALLOWED IN LARGE AMOUNTS.

Storage

Store in a cool and dry place.

EXPERIMENT 57

Zinc Sulphate and Zinc Chloride Mouthwash BPC

Aim

To prepare and submit 20 ml of Zinc Sulphate and Zinc Chloride mouthwash.

Synonym

Collutorium Zinci Sulphatis et Chloridi.

Formula

Sl.No	Ingredients	Official formula	Working formula
1	Zinc Sulphate	20 g	
2	Zinc Chloride	10 g	
3	Dilute hydrochloric acid	10 ml	
4	Compound Tartrazine solution	10 ml	
5	Chloroform water	500 ml	
6	Purified water (q.s)	1000 ml	

Principle

Mouthwashes are medicated liquids, which are used to clean and deodorize the buccal cavity. They are pleasant in taste and odour. They are formulated either in ready to use form or as concentrated preparations. If they are dispensed in concentrated form, they are required to be diluted before use.

In the following preparation, Zinc Sulphate and Zinc Chloride are used for their astringent properties. Compound Tartrazine solution is the colouring agent. Chloroform water flavours the preparation.

Procedure

1. Zinc Sulphate and Zinc Chloride were dissolved in a small quantity of purified water.

2. Dilute hydrochloric acid was added to the solution.

3. Compound Tartrazine solution and chloroform water were added.

4. Purified water was added to produce the required volume.

Category

Astringent.

Direction

Dilute 1 ml of the mouthwash with 20 ml of warm water before use.

Auxiliary label

FOR EXTERNAL USE ONLY.

NOT TO BE TAKEN.

NOT TO BE SWALLOWED IN LARGE AMOUNTS.

Storage

Store in a cool and dry place.

Chlorhexidine Gluconate Mouthwash

Aim

To prepare and submit 20 ml of Chlorhexidine Gluconate mouthwash.

Formula

Sl.No	Ingredients	Official formula	Working formula
1	Chlorhexidine gluconate	0.12 g	
2	Ethanol (95%)	11 ml	
3	Sorbitol	5 g	
4	Glycerol	2.5 ml	
5	Peppermint oil	1 ml	
6	FD&C blue no. 1	q.s	
7	Purified water (q.s)	100 ml	

Principle

Mouthwashes are medicated liquids, which are used to clean and deodorize the buccal cavity. They are pleasant in taste and odour. They are formulated either in ready to use form or as concentrated preparations. If they are dispensed in concentrated form, they are required to be diluted before use.

In the following preparation, Chlorhexidine gluconate acts as an antibacterial. This preparation can be used as a dental rinse for treatment of gingivitis, promote gum healing after dental surgery, control mouth ulcers and for maintaining oral hygiene.

Ethanol is used to solubilize the oil. Glycerol is a sweetener and humectants. Sorbitol is also a sweetener and humectant and Peppermint oil is the flavouring agent.

Procedure

1. Chlorhexidine gluconate was dissolved in a small quantity of purified water.

2. Glycerol and Sorbitol were added to the solution.

3. Peppermint oil was dissolved in ethanol and added to the above solution. Required amount of colour was added.

4. Purified water was added to produce the required volume.

Category

Antibacterial.

Direction

Swish for 30 seconds with 15 ml (one capful) of undiluted oral rinse after brushing, then expectorate; repeat twice daily (morning and evening).

Auxiliary label

FOR EXTERNAL USE ONLY.

NOT TO BE TAKEN.

NOT TO BE SWALLOWED IN LARGE AMOUNTS.

Storage

Store in a cool and dry place away from light.

EXPERIMENT 59

Phenol Gargle BPC

Aim

To prepare and submit 20 ml of Phenol Gargle.

Synonym

Carbolic acid gargle.

Gargarisma Phenolis.

Formula

Sl.No	Ingredients	Official formula	Working formula
1	Phenol Glycerin	50 ml	
2	Amaranth solution	10 ml	
3	Purified water (q.s)	1000 ml	

Preparation of Phenol glycerin

Phenol	16 g
Glycerin	84 g

Dissolve the phenol in glycerin with the aid of gentle heat if necessary.

(Glycerin is added to reduce the causticity of phenol. Dilution with water renders Phenol glycerin caustic; hence the preparation may be diluted with glycerin if necessary).

Principle

Phenol gargle is used as an anti- bacterial in the treatment of pharynx and nasopharynx infections. Glycerin is used to increase the viscosity of the preparation and also gives a sweet taste to the preparation. Amaranth solution is used as the colouring agent.

Procedure

1. Weighed quantities of glycerin and phenol were mixed together to prepare phenol glycerin.

2. The required quantity of phenol glycerin was mixed with amaranth solution and made up to volume with purified water.

Category

Antibacterial.

Direction

Dilute with an equal volume of warm water before use.

Auxiliary label

NOT TO BE TAKEN.

NOT TO BE SWALLOWED IN LARGE AMOUNTS.

PROLONGED USE SHOULD BE AVOIDED.

Storage

Store in a cool and dry place.

EXPERIMENT 60

Potassium Permanganate Gargle BPC

Aim

To prepare and submit 20 ml of Potassium Permanganate Gargle.

Formula

Sl.No	Ingredients	Official formula	Working formula
1	Potassium Permanganate solution	10 ml	
2	Purified water (q.s)	1000 ml	

Principle

Gargles are aqueous solutions used to prevent or treat throat infections. They are bought into intimate contact with the mucous membranes of the throat and are allowed to remain there for a few seconds before they are thrown out of the mouth.

Procedure

1. Potassium Permanganate solution was mixed with a small quantity of water and shaken well.

2. Purified water was added to produce the required volume.

Category

Antiseptic.

Direction

Mix with water and use as a gargle.

Auxiliary label

NOT TO BE TAKEN.

NOT TO BE SWALLOWED IN LARGE AMOUNTS.

PROLONGED USE SHOULD BE AVOIDED.

Storage

Store in a cool and dry place.

EXPERIMENT 61

Povidone- Iodine Gargle

Aim

To prepare and submit 20 ml of Povidone-Iodine Gargle.

Formula

Sl.No	Ingredients	Official formula	Working formula
1	Povidone-Iodine	1 g	
2	Ethanol (95%)	8.5 ml	
3	Glycerol	5 ml	
4	Saccharin Sodium	0.1 g	
5	Purified water (q.s)	100 ml	

Principle

Gargles are aqueous solutions used to prevent or treat throat infections. They are bought into intimate contact with the mucous membranes of the throat and are allowed to remain there for a few seconds before they are thrown out of the mouth.

This medicated gargle contains povidone-iodine, a multivalent broad spectrum local antiseptic having bactericidal and fungicidal properties. Povidone - Iodine is a complex polymer of iodine with polyvinyl pyrrolidone (a high-molecular weight, water soluble polymer), a complex that enhances the bactericidal activity of iodine. Iodine is slowly released from the complex, providing antimicrobial action. Moreover Iodine carriers decrease the free available iodine and therefore minimize the side effects of elemental iodine. The gargle is non-irritating to the oral mucous membrane and non-staining to the teeth or denture. The gargle is recommended for relief of painful infections and inflammatory conditions of the mouth and pharynx, and can also be used as a routine mouthwash.

Procedure

1. Povidone Iodine was dissolved in a small quantity of purified water.
2. Ethanol, glycerol and saccharin sodium were added.
3. Purified water was added to produce the required volume.

Category

Antiseptic.

Direction

Use the gargle undiluted for 30 seconds.

Repeat every 3- 4 hours.

Auxiliary label

NOT TO BE TAKEN.

NOT TO BE SWALLOWED IN LARGE AMOUNTS.

PROLONGED USE SHOULD BE AVOIDED.

Storage

Store in a cool and dry place away from light.

Marketed Formulations

BETADINE

DIFFLAM

Throat Paints

Paints are liquid preparations for application to the skin or mucous surfaces. They usually contain drugs with antiseptic, astringent or analgesic properties.

Throat paints are used for mouth and throat infections. Throat paints are viscous in nature due to a high content of glycerin, which also helps the preparation to remain in contact with the affected site for a longer period of time.

E.g. Compound Iodine Paint (Mandl's Paint)

Paints are usually applied with a brush.

Auxiliary Label

FOR EXTERNAL USE ONLY.

NOT TO BE TAKEN.

NOT TO BE SWALLOWED IN LARGE AMOUNTS.

Containers

Throat Paints are supplied in coloured wide mouthed containers. A soft brush may be supplied along with the preparation.

Marketed Formulations

SG PAINT (Centaur)

SENSOFORM GUM PAINT (Indoco)

EXPERIMENT 62

Compound
Iodine Paint BPC

Aim

To prepare and submit 20 ml of Compound Iodine Paint.

Synonym

Mandl's Paint.

Formula

Sl.No	Ingredients	Official formula	Working formula
1	Potassium iodide	25 g	
2	Iodine	12.5 g	
3	Alcohol (90%)	40 ml	
4	Water	25 ml	
5	Peppermint Oil	4 ml	
6	Glycerin (q.s)	1000 ml	

Principle

Compound iodine Paint or Mandl's paint is a throat paint used in the treatment of Pharyngitis and Tonsilitis. Glycerin is used as the vehicle as it is viscous and adheres to the mucous membranes of the throat for a long time. This preparation should be applied with a fine camel hair brush

Procedure

1. Potassium iodide was dissolved in water.

2. Iodine was added to it and stirred until it dissolved completely.

3. Peppermint oil dissolved in alcohol and a small portion of glycerin was added.

4. Sufficient glycerin was added to produce the required volume and mixed.

5. The required quantity of phenol glycerin was mixed with amaranth solution and made up to volume with purified water.

Category

Antiseptic and Astringent.

Direction

Apply with a brush.

Auxiliary label

NOT TO BE TAKEN.

NOT TO BE SWALLOWED IN LARGE AMOUNTS.

SHAKE WELL BEFORE USE (because some of the oil separates on storage).

Storage

Store in a cool and dry place. Protect from light.

Enemas

Enemas are aqueous or oily solutions or suspensions that are introduced into the rectum for cleansing, therapeutic or diagnostic purposes. Enemas can be broadly classified into two types:

1. ***Evacuation enemas (Cleansing enemas):*** are preparations employed to cleanse the bowel (as in the case of constipation or before an operation).The volume of evacuant enemas may be as much as one litre and should be warmed to body temperature before use. If the enema is too cold, intestinal cramping may occur and if it is too hot, it may damage the intestinal mucosa. They act by any one the following mechanisms:

   (a) By stimulating peristalsis – due to their large volume (e.g. plain water) or by causing osmotic retention of water in the bowel (e.g. Sodium phosphate enema)

   (b) By lubricating impacted faeces – e.g. Arachis oil enema

2. ***Retention enemas :*** are used for local or systemic effects and their volume do not 100ml. Retention enemas are used to administer anthelmintics (quassia- for thread worms), anti-inflammatory agents (corticosteroids for ulcerative colitis), sedatives (chloral hydrate, paraldehyde), nutrients and Barium sulphate enema(used for X-ray examination of the lower bowel).

Auxiliary Label

FOR RECTAL USE ONLY.

TO BE WARMED TO BODY TEMPERATURE BEFORE USE.

Containers

Enemas should be packed in colour, fluted, screw capped glass bottles. They are also available in plastic squeeze bags with a rectal nozzle.

EXPERIMENT 63

Glycerin Enema

Aim

To prepare and submit 20 ml of Glycerin enema.

Formula

Sl.No	Ingredients	Standard formula	Working formula
1	Glycerin	50 ml	
2	Warm water (q.s)	1000 ml	

Principle

Enemas are aqueous or oily preparations that are meant for rectal administration for cleansing, therapeutic or diagnostic purposes.

The following precautions are to be taken while administering enemas.

1. The enema solution should be warmed to body temperature before administration. If the enema is too hot, it may damage the intestinal mucosa and if it is too cold, intestinal cramping may occur.

2. The patient should lie on the side, the lower leg extended and the upper leg flexed towards the chest.

3. The end of the enema tube should be lubricated with a water-soluble lubricant.

181

4. The enema tube should be inserted with a twisting motion. It should not be inserted more than 7.5- 15 cm.

5. The patient should take a deep breath, which facilitate the procedure.

6. While administering large volumes of cleansing enema, the enema bag should not be hung more than 30cm above the rectum because increased pressure results in severe cramping and could rupture the intestinal wall.

7. Check any obstruction in the line.

8. Small volume retention enemas are given slowly by squeezing the enema bottle. It should not be given more than 180ml at a time.

    In glycerin in enema, glycerin acts as a stimulant laxative. It stimulates the rectal mucosa and promotes defecation. It also lubricates and softens the faecal matter.

Procedure

Glycerin was mixed with warm water and made up to volume.

Category

Stimulant laxative.

Auxiliary label

FOR RECTAL USE ONLY.

TO BE WARMED TO BODY TEMPERATURE BEFORE USE.

Storage

Store in a cool and dry place.

Inhalations

Inhalations are liquid preparations composed of or containing volatile ingredients, which when vaporized in a suitable manner, are intended to be brought into contact with the lining of the respiratory tract. They are used to relieve congestion and inflammation of the respiratory tract.

The ingredients are volatile at room temperature and may be inhaled from a handkerchief or an absorbent pad on which they have been placed. They can also be added to hot, but not boiling water and the vapour inhaled for five to ten minutes.

Auxiliary Label

FOR EXTERNAL USE ONLY.

Direction

Add 5 ml of the inhalation to 500 ml of hot water and inhale the vapour.

Containers

Inhalations should be dispensed in white fluted bottles.

Marketed Formulation

KARVOL PLUS INHALANT (Indoco Remedies).

EXPERIMENT 64

Benzoin Inhalation BPC

Aim

To prepare and submit 20 ml of Benzoin Inhalation.

Synonym

Vapor Benzoini.

Formula

Sl.No	Ingredients	Official formula	Working formula
1	Benzoin, crushed	100 g	
2	Prepared Storax	50 g	
3	Alcohol-95% (q.s)	1000 ml	

Principle

Inhalations are liquid preparations containing volatile ingredients and are used to relieve congestion and inflammation of the respiratory tract.

Inhalations may be placed on an absorbent pad or handkerchief and inhaled. The vapours can also be inhaled by adding a few drops to hot water.

Benzoin is a balsamic resin obtained form the incised stem of *Styrax benzoin* and *Styrax paralleloneurus* and is commonly known as Sumathra benzoin.

Procedure

1. Benzoin and Prepared storax were macerated together with 750 ml of alcohol for twenty four hours.

2. The mixture was then filtered and sufficient alcohol was passed through the filter to produce the required volume.

Category

In the treatment of chronic rhinitis (inflammation of the nasal mucous membranes).

Direction

Add 5 ml of the inhalation to 500 ml of hot water and inhale the vapour.

Auxiliary label

FOR EXTERNAL USE ONLY.

Storage

Store in a cool and dry place.

EXPERIMENT 65

Menthol Inhalation BPC

Aim

To prepare and submit 20 ml of Menthol Inhalation.

Formula

Sl.No	Ingredients	Official formula	Working formula
1	Menthol	0.5 g	
2	Methylated Spirit (q.s)	50 ml	

Principle

Inhalations are liquid preparations containing volatile ingredients and are used to relieve congestion and inflammation of the respiratory tract.

Inhalations may be placed on an absorbent pad or handkerchief and inhaled. The vapours can also be inhaled by adding a few drops to hot water.

Procedure

1. Menthol was dissolved in a small quantity of Methylated spirit.

2. Sufficient methylated spirit was added to produce the required volume.

Category

Nasal Decongestant.

Direction

Add 5 ml of the inhalation to 500 ml of hot water and inhale the vapour.

Auxiliary label

FOR EXTERNAL USE ONLY.

Storage

Store in a cool and dry place. Protect from light.

EXPERIMENT 66

Menthol and Eucalyptus Inhalation BPC

Aim

To prepare and submit 20 ml of Menthol and Eucalyptus Inhalation.

Synonym

Vapor Mentholis et Eucalypti.

Formula

Sl.No	Ingredients	Official formula	Working formula
1	Eucalyptus oil	100 ml	
2	Light magnesium carbonate	70 g	
3	Menthol	20 g	
4	Purified water (q.s)	1000 ml	

Principle

Aqueous Inhalations consist of one or more volatile oils in water. To ensure uniform dispersion of the oils on shaking, light Magnesium Carbonate is added to absorb some of the oil and finely subdivide the remainder.

Procedure

1. Menthol was finely powdered in a glass mortar.

2. Eucalyptus oil was added and stirred until the solid dissolved completely.

3. Light magnesium Carbonate was added in small amounts and mixed well.

4. Sufficient water was added to produce the required volume.

Category

Nasal Decongestant.

Direction

Add one teaspoonful to a pint of hot, but not boiling water and inhale the vapour.

(Use of boiling water will vaporize the ingredients too quickly and cause discomfort to the patient).

Auxiliary label

FOR EXTERNAL USE ONLY.

Storage

Store in a cool and dry place. Protect from light.

Marketed Formulation

KARVOL PLUS INHALANT (Indoco Remedies).

Semisolid Dosage Forms

1. OINTMENTS

Ointments are semisolid preparations meant for external application to the skin or mucous membranes. They usually contain a medicament / medicaments dissolved, suspended or emulsified in an ointment base.

They are greasy in nature. The bases used in the preparation of ointments are hydrocarbon bases, absorption bases, emulsifying bases and water soluble bases.

E.g Diclofenac Sodium Ointment.

Auxiliary Label

FOR EXTERNAL USE ONLY.

Containers

Ointments are supplied in collapsible tubes or wide mouthed containers (as in the case of Non- Staining Iodine Ointment BPC).

Marketed Formulations

DIPROVATE –G (Fulford)

NEOSPORIN-H (GSK)

TOPCORT (Cipla)

2. PASTES

Pastes are semisolid preparations intended for external application to the skin. They are generally thick and stiff due to the presence of a large amount (50%) of finely powdered solids. When applied to the skin, they adhere well, forming a thick coat that protects and soothes inflamed or itchy skin. They do not melt at ordinary temperature and thus form a protective coating over the area where they are applied.

Because of their powder content, pastes are porous and can help perspiration to escape. They are emollient but less greasy than ointments.

E.g. Compound Zinc Paste.

Auxiliary Label

FOR EXTERNAL USE ONLY.

Containers

Pastes are supplied in wide mouthed containers.

3. POULTICES

Poultices are paste like preparations used externally to reduce inflammation. They are intended to supply warmth to inflamed parts of the body.

E.g. Kaolin poultice BPC.

Before application, the poultice is heated with occasional stirring until it can be tolerated on the back of the hand. Then it is spread thickly on lint or any other dressing and applied to the affected area.

Auxiliary Label

FOR EXTERNAL USE ONLY.

Containers

Poultices can be supplied in wide mouthed containers or in tin containers that withstand heating in water.

4. JELLIES

Jellies are transparent or translucent, non- greasy, semisolid gels, generally applied externally.

They are used for medication, lubrication and other applications like patch testing of allergens and ECG testing.

E.g. Kaolin poultice BPC.

Auxiliary Label

FOR EXTERNAL USE ONLY.

Containers

Jellies are supplied in collapsible tubes or wide mouthed containers.

5. CREAMS

Creams are semi solid preparations intended for application to the skin or mucous membranes. They may be water in oil (oily creams) or oil in water (aqueous creams).

E.g. Cold cream.

Auxiliary Label

FOR EXTERNAL USE ONLY.

Containers

Creams should be dispensed in well closed containers to prevent evaporation of the aqueous phase. Collapsible tubes or wide mouthed plastic containers are preferred.

Marketed Formulations

TOPCORT (Cipla).

EXPERIMENT 67

Kaolin Poultice BPC

Aim

To prepare and submit 20 g Kaolin Poultice (Calculate 5g extra).

Synonym

Cataplasma Kaolini.

Formula

Sl. No	Ingredients	Official formula	Batch formula	Working formula (for 5g extra)
1	Heavy Kaolin (dried at 100°C and finely sifted)	56.5 g		
2	Boric acid (finely sifted)	4.5 g		
3	Thymol	0.05 g		
4	Peppermint oil	0.05 ml		
5	Methyl Salicylate	0.2 ml		
6	Glycerin	38.7 g		

Principle

Poultices are paste like preparations used externally to reduce inflammation because they retain heat well. They are intended to supply warmth to inflamed parts of the body.

Kaolin poultice is a thick paste with good heat capacity.

Heavy kaolin is used as it can retain heat well. Since Kaolin is obtained from mineral origin, it may be contaminated with spores of *Clostridium tetanii, Clostridium welchii* and *Bacillus anthracis*. Therefore it must be sterilized by heating at 160°C for 1 hour before use.

The preparation also contains glycerol which is hygroscopic in nature and can draw infected material from the tissues when the poultice is used fro boils and infections.

Boric acid is a weak antimicrobial agent.

Thymol is a powerful bactericide.

Peppermint oil perfumes the preparation.

Methyl Salicylate is an anti-rheumatic drug.

Before application, the poultice is heated with occasional stirring until it can be tolerated on the back of the hand. Then it is spread thickly on lint or any other dressing and applied to the affected area.

Kaolin Poultice should be stored in well closed containers to prevent loss of volatile ingredients and absorption of moisture from the atmosphere by glycerin.

Procedure

1. Kaolin and boric acid were taken into a mortar and mixed thoroughly.

2. Glycerin was added to the powder mixture and triturated until a smooth paste was formed.

3. The paste was heated at 120°C for 1 hour in a hot air oven, with occasional stirring. (Heating is done to destroy microbes that may be present in Kaolin. The temperature is limited to 120°C to prevent decomposition of glycerin).

4. The paste was cooled and the remaining ingredients were added and stirred thoroughly.

5. The paste was then packed into air tight containers to prevent absorption of moisture by the glycerol and loss of volatile constituents.

Category

Anti-inflammatory and Counter -irritant.

Direction

Spread the warm poultice on a dressing and apply on the affected part.

Auxiliary label

FOR EXTERNAL USE ONLY.

Storage

Store in a cool and dry place.

Zinc Gelatin Jelly BPC

Aim

To prepare and submit 20 g of Zinc Gelatin Jelly. (Calculate 5g extra).

Synonym

Unna's Paste.

Formula

Sl. No	Ingredients	Official formula	Batch formula	Working formula (for 5g extra)
1	Zinc Oxide	15 g		
2	Gelatin	15 g		
3	Glycerol	35g		
4	Water	35 g		

Principle

Jellies are transparent or translucent, non- greasy, semisolid gels, generally applied externally.

They are used for medication, lubrication and other applications like patch testing of allergens and ECG testing.

Jellies can be made stiff by the addition of 15% gelatin. Such jellies are melted before use and after cooling to the desired temperature, applied with a soft brush to the affected area. The area is bandaged and further layers of jelly and bandage is applied.

Procedure

1. Glycerol was heated to 100°C.

2. Gelatin was soaked in water.

3. Hot glycerol was added to gelatin, stirred well and transferred a boiling water bath. Heating was continued until the gelatin melts completely.

4. The glycerol-gelatin base was then heated at 100°C for 1 hour to destroy microbes present in gelatin.

5. Zinc Oxide was then added in small amounts to the molten base, with continuous stirring, until it is completely suspended.

6. The mass was then poured into a tray to a depth of about 1 cm and allowed to cool.

7. Once cooled, it was cut into pieces of about 1.5 cm^2 and packed in wide mouth containers.

Category

Antiseptic.

Direction

Melt the pieces. On cooling, apply on the affected area with a soft brush. Cover with a bandage.

Auxiliary label

FOR EXTERNAL USE ONLY.

Storage

Store in a cool and dry place.

Sodium Alginate Jelly

Aim

To prepare and submit 20 g of Sodium Alginate Jelly. (Calculate 5g extra).

Formula

Sl. No	Ingredients	Standard formula	Batch formula	Working formula (for 5g extra)
1	Sodium Alginate	7 g		
2	Glycerol	7 g		
3	Methyl Paraben	0.2 g		
4	Calcium Gluconate	0.05 g		
5	Purified Water (q.s)	100 g		

Principle

The following preparation is a jelly base made with Sodium alginate.

Sodium Alginate jellies may be used as dermatological vehicles (5-10%) and lubricants (1.5 – 2%).

Calcium gluconate is added to increase the viscosity of the jelly and glycerol helps to disperse the alginate.

Since glycerol is hygroscopic in nature, it prevents drying out of the preparation, during its storage. If the jelly is to be used on the skin, then glycerol will provide a humectant effect and keep the skin moist.

Methyl paraben is the preservative.

This base should be stored overnight before use.

Procedure

1. Sodium alginate was wetted with the glycerol in glass mortar.

2. Methyl paraben and Calcium gluconate were dissolved in about 80 ml of water by heating.

3. The mixture was cooled to 60°C and stirred rapidly with a high speed stirrer.

4. The sodium alginate – glycerol mixture was added in small quantities to the Calcium gluconate solution, with continuous stirring until a homogenous dispersion was obtained.

5. Purified water was added to produce the required weight.

Category

Jelly base.

Lubricant for catheters, gloves, electrodiagnostic equipment.

Auxiliary label

FOR EXTERNAL USE ONLY.

Storage

Store in a cool and dry place.

EXPERIMENT 70

Lubricating Jelly

Aim

To prepare and submit 20 g of Lubricating jelly. (Calculate 5g extra).

Formula

Sl. No	Ingredients	Official formula	Batch formula	Working formula (for 5g extra)
1	Sodium Carboxymethylcellulose	5 g		
2	Glycerol	15 g		
3	Methyl Paraben	0.1 g		
4	Patent Blue	0.001 g		
5	Purified Water (q.s)	100 g		

Principle

The following preparation is a jelly base made with a cellulose ether base.

Sodium Carboxymethylcellulose (SCMC) is use as a jelling agent for dermatological vehicles (5%) and lubricants (1.5 – 5%).

SCMC is easier to dissolve in water and its mucilage is clear in nature.

Glycerol is added to prevent drying of the preparation, during its storage. If the jelly is to be used on the skin, then glycerol will provide a humectant effect and keep the skin moist.

Methyl paraben is the preservative.

Patent blue is the colouring agent.

Procedure

1. Methyl paraben was dissolved in a small quantity of water by heating.

2. The solution was cooled and stirred rapidly with a high speed stirrer.

3. SCMC was wetted with the glycerol in glass mortar.

4. The SCMC – glycerol mixture was added in small quantities to the Methyl paraben solution, with continuous stirring until a clear gel was obtained.

5. Patent blue solution was added to the gel.

6. Purified water was added to produce the required weight.

Category

Jelly base.

Lubricant for catheters, gloves, electrodiagnostic equipment.

Auxiliary label

FOR EXTERNAL USE ONLY.

Storage

Store in a cool and dry place.

EXPERIMENT 71

Simple Ointment BP

Aim

To prepare and submit 20 g of Simple ointment. (Calculate 5g extra).

Formula

Sl. No	Ingredients	Official formula	Batch formula	Working formula (for 5g extra)
1	Wool fat (Anhydrous)	50 g		
2	Hard paraffin	50 g		
3	Cetostearyl alcohol	50 g		
4	White / Yellow Soft Paraffin (q.s)	1000g		

Principle

Ointments are semisolid preparations meant for external application to the skin or mucous membranes. They usually contain a medicament / medicaments dissolved, suspended or emulsified in an ointment base.

Simple ointment is an ointment made with an absorption base. Absorption bases are hydrophillic and can absorb considerable amounts of water or aqueous solutions.

In the following preparation, Wool fat (Anhydrous Lanolin) is a non - emulsified absorption base that can absorb about 50% of its weight of water to form a W/O emulsion.

Hard Paraffin is used to harden the preparation.

Cetostearyl alcohol is used as an emulsion stabilizer and white/yellow soft paraffin is the ointment base.

Procedure

1. Weighed quantities of Wool fat, hard paraffin, Cetostearyl alcohol and soft paraffin were melted in a china dish at 70°C and stirred well until it solidified.

2. The ointment was then packed in aluminium collapsible tubes.

Category

Ointment base.

Emollient.

Auxiliary label

FOR EXTERNAL USE ONLY.

Storage

Store in a cool and dry place.

Sulphur Ointment BP

Aim

To prepare and submit 20 g of Sulphur ointment (Calculate 5g extra).

Formula

Sl. No	Ingredients	Official formula	Batch formula	Working formula (for 5g extra)
1	Sublimed sulphur	10 g		
2	Simple ointment (q.s)	100 g		

Principle

Sulphur ointment is an epidermic ointment meant for local action on the epidermis. Sulphur Ointment contains Sulphur, which is used for Bacterial infections, inflammatory skin disorders, parasitic infections, acne and other skin conditions. Sulphur probably reduces sebaceous gland activity and hence used in the treatment of acne.

Simple ointment is the ointment base.

Procedure

1. Sublimed sulphur was triturated and the required quantity was transferred to an ointment slab.

2. It was then blended with simple ointment in geometric proportion.

3. The ointment was then filled into ointment tubes and sealed.

Category

Keratolytic.

Treatment of Scabies, Acne and Seborrheic Dermatitis.

Direction

Apply a thin layer on the affected area.

Auxiliary label

FOR EXTERNAL USE ONLY.

Storage

Store in a cool and dry place.

Note

(Sulphur ointment can also be prepared with 10%w/w of Precipitated Sulphur).

Non Staining Iodine Ointment with Methyl Salicylate BPC

Aim

To prepare and submit 20 g of Non staining iodine ointment with Methyl Salicylate. (Calculate 5g extra).

Formula

Sl. No	Ingredients	Official formula	Batch formula	Working formula (for 5g extra)
1	Iodine	5 g		
2	Arachis oil	15 g		
3	Methyl Salicylate	2 ml		
4	Yellow soft Paraffin	78 g		

Principle

Non- Staining Iodine ointment is prepared by chemical reaction.

Arachis oil is an unsaturated fatty acid. Iodine gets trapped in the unsaturated linkage to form a complex and the linkage gets saturated. As the iodine forms a complex with the oil, it is not in the free state and loses its staining property. The product is greenish black, but leaves no stain when rubbed into the skin. Hence they are called non-staining iodine ointment.

Procedure

1. Iodine was finely powdered in a glass mortar and the required quantity was weighed and added to Arachis oil taken in a glass flask and stirred well.

2. The mixture was heated on a water bath at 50°C, stirring occasionally. Heating was continued until the colour of the mixture changed from brown to greenish black. This process will take several hours.

3. The soft paraffin was warmed to 40°C. The iodised oil was added to it and mixed well.

4. The mixture was removed from heat.

5. The contents were stirred until it cooled and Methyl salicylate was added.

6. The ointment was then filled into light resistant, wide mouth containers.

Category

Topical analgesic and anti-inflammatory.

Direction

Rub on the affected part.

Auxiliary label

FOR EXTERNAL USE ONLY.

NOT TO BE APPLIED ON BROKEN SKIN.

Storage

Store in a cool and dry place. Protect from light.

Methyl Salicylate Ointment BPC

Aim

To prepare and submit 20 g of Methyl Salicylate ointment (Calculate 5g extra).

Synonym

Unguentum Methylis Salicylatis Forte.

Formula

Sl. No	Ingredients	Official formula	Batch formula	Working formula (for 5g extra)
1	Methyl Salicylate	500 g		
2	Hydrous wool fat	250 g		
3	White bees wax	250 g		

Principle

Ointments are semisolid preparations meant for external application to the skin or mucous membranes. They usually contain a medicament / medicaments dissolved, suspended or emulsified in an ointment base.

Methyl salicylate ointment is an ointment made with an absorption base. Absorption bases are hydrophillic and can absorb considerable amounts of water or aqueous solutions.

Hydrous Wool fat (Lanolin) is prepared from wool fat (70%) and water (30%). They are categorized as W/O emulsions that are capable of absorbing more water.

White beeswax is used to stiffen the preparation.

Methyl salicylate (wintergreen oil) has counter irritant properties and is used as an anti- rheumatic drug.

Procedure

1. Hydrous wool fat and White bees wax were melted together.

2. Methyl Salicylate was added to the molten mass, with stirring.

3. The ointment was stirred well until it cooled.

4. The ointment was then transferred to wide mouth containers.

Category

Counter- irritant.

Direction

To be applied on the affected area with rubbing.

Auxiliary label

FOR EXTERNAL USE ONLY.

Storage

Store in a cool and dry place.

Bentonite Gel

Aim

To prepare and submit 20 g of Bentonite Gel (Calculate 5g extra).

Formula

Sl. No	Ingredients	Official formula	Batch formula	Working formula (for 5g extra)
1	Zinc Oxide	10 g		
2	Glycerol	10 g		
3	Bentonite	10 g		
4	Purified water	qs 100 g		

Principle

Gels containing 7-20% of bentonite are used as dermatological bases. They are opalescent and lack the attractive clear appearance like other gels. The residue left behind on the skin is powdery with a silky finish. Bentonite should be sterilized for preparations applied to open wounds. Zinc oxide is an antiseptic. 10% Glycerol is used as a humectant and to impart a moist residue.

Procedure

1. Finely sifted zinc oxide was mixed with bentonite in a mortar.

2.   The mixture was then triturated with glycerol.

3.   Water was then added in small quantities with constant sirring.

Category

Antiseptic.

Direction

To be applied on the affected area.

Auxiliary label

FOR EXTERNAL USE ONLY.

NOT TO BE APPLIED ON OPEN WOUNDS.

Storage

Store in a cool and dry place.

EXPERIMENT 76

Cold Cream

Aim

To prepare and submit 20 g of Cold Cream. (Calculate 5g extra).

Formula

Sl. No	Ingredients	Standard formula	Batch formula	Working formula (for 5g extra)
1	White beeswax	10 g		
2	Liquid Paraffin	30 g		
3	Borax	0.5 g		
4	Water	9.5 ml		
5	Perfume	q.s		

Principle

Cold cream is a W/O emulsion as the amount of oil predominates. When applied to the skin, a cooling effect is produced due to the slow evaporation of water contained in the emulsion.

The soap formed by interaction between beeswax and borax acts as the emulsifying agent for the cream.

Cold cream is used for its emollient and protective properties.

Procedure

1. Beeswax was melted with liquid paraffin to a temperature of 70°C.

2. Borax was dissolved in water and heated to 70°C.

3. The borax solution was added slowly to the molten mixture and stirred rapidly until the cream cooled.

4. The perfume was added.

5. The cream was then filled into wide mouth containers and closed tightly.

Category

Protective and emollient.

Auxiliary label

FOR EXTERNAL USE ONLY.

Storage

Store in a cool and dry place.

Marketed Formulations

PONDS (Cold cream)

AYUR (Cold cream)

Vanishing Cream

Aim

To prepare and submit 20 g of Vanishing Cream. (Calculate 5g extra).

Synonym

Foundation cream.

Formula

Sl. No	Ingredients	Standard formula	Batch formula	Working formula (for 5g extra)
1	Stearic acid	15 g		
2	Water	76.3 ml		
3	Glycerin	8 g		
4	Potassium hydroxide	0.7 g		
5	Perfume	q.s		

Principle

Vanishing creams are creams that spread easily and disappear when rubbed on the skin. They are also called foundation creams as they can be applied to the skin to provide a smooth emollient base before the application of face powder and other make up preparations.

In this preparation, part of the stearic acid is saponified by Potassium hydroxide to form the soap. The soap thus formed saponifies the remaining stearic acid.

Vanishing cream is a O/W emulsion as the main constituent is water.

Glycerin is used for its humectant properties.

Procedure

1. Stearic acid was melted on a water bath to 70°C.

2. Potassium hydroxide was dissolved in water, glycerin was added and the mixture was heated to 70°C.

3. The potassium hydroxide solution was added slowly to the molten stearic acid with constant stirring.

4. Once the cream cooled, the perfume was added.

5. The cream was then filled into wide mouth containers and closed tightly.

Category

Foundation cream.

Auxiliary label

FOR EXTERNAL USE ONLY.

Storage

Store in a cool and dry place.

Marketed Formulations

PONDS (Vanishing cream).

EXPERIMENT 78

Compound Zinc Paste BP

Aim

To prepare and submit 20 g of Compound Zinc Paste BP (Calculate 5g extra).

Synonym

Zinc Paste.

Formula

Sl. No	Ingredients	Official formula	Batch formula	Working formula (for 5g extra)
1	Zinc oxide			
2	Starch			
3	White Soft Paraffin (q.s)			

Principle

Pastes are semisolid preparations intended for external application to the skin. They are generally thick and stiff due to the presence of a large amount (50%) of finely powdered solids. When applied to the skin, they adhere well, forming a thick coat that protects and soothes inflamed or itchy skin. They do not melt at ordinary temperature and thus form a protective coating over the area where they are applied.

Because of their powder content, pastes are porous and can help perspiration to escape. They are emollient but less greasy than ointments.

In the following preparation, soft paraffin is used as the base. Zinc oxide has antiseptic properties.

Compound Zinc Paste can be used for a variety of dermatological conditions, including eczema and psoriasis.

Procedure

1. Zinc oxide and starch were sifted through sieve no.180, separately and weighed.

2. White soft paraffin was melted using minimum heat.

3. The molten base was added in small amounts to the powders, with continuous trituration until a smooth paste was obtained.

4. Mixing was continued until the preparation became cold.

5. The paste was then packed into a suitable wide mouth container.

Category

Antiseptic.

Direction

Spread the paste thickly on white lint and apply to the affected area.

Auxiliary label

FOR EXTERNAL USE ONLY.

Storage

Store in a cool and dry place.

Diclofenac Gel

Aim

To prepare and submit 20 g of Diclofenac gel (Calculate 5g extra).

Formula

Sl. No	Ingredients	Official formula	Batch formula	Working formula (for 5g extra)
1	Diclofenac Sodium	1.2 g		
2	Carbopol 940	1 g		
3	Triethanolamine	3.1 ml		
4	Propylene Glycol	12 ml		
5	Diethyl Phthalate	1 ml		
6	Perfume	0.6 ml		
7	Purified water (q.s)	100 g		

Principle

Gels are semisolid systems consisting of either suspensions made up of small inorganic particles or large organic molecules interpenetrated by a liquid. In the following preparation, Diclofenac Sodium is a Nonsteroidal anti-inflammatory drug (NSAID) used for the relief of osteoarthritis pain, pain due to skeletal muscle, relief of the pain of osteoarthritis of knees and hands, bone fractures and other conditions.

Carbopol 940 is the gelling agent and forms a sparkling clear gel. Triethanolamine is used as the neutralizing agent for Carbopol 940. Propylene glycol is a humectant, improves the consistency of the gel and helps in easy extrudability from the tube.

Procedure

1. Weighed quantity of carbopol was dispersed in half the quantity of water and allowed to soak for 1 hr.

2. Triethanolamine was added drop wise with continuous stirring to obtain gel like consistency.

3. Diclofenac sodium was dissolved in propylene glycol and added to the gel.

4. Diethyl phthalate and perfume were also added.

5. The gel was made up to the required weight with water, blended uniformly and filled into collapsible tubes.

Category

Anti-inflammatory.

Direction

As directed by the physician.

Auxiliary label

FOR EXTERNAL USE ONLY.

Storage

Store in a cool and dry place.

Marketed Formulations

ENAC gel

VOLTAREN

DICLOC

Ear Drops

Ear drops are solutions and suspensions of medicaments in water, glycerol dilute alcohol, propylene glycol or any other suitable solvent, for instillation into the ear.

They contain medicaments for

> Treating mild infections (E.g. Chloramphenicol)

> Softening wax (E.g Hydrogen Peroxide)

> Cleaning after infections (E.g Spirit)

> Anesthetics (E.g Phenol)

The vehicle is usually water but glycerol may be included for its softening effect on wax. The high viscosity of glycerol helps in adherence to infected surfaces.

Auxiliary Label

FOR EXTERNAL USE ONLY.

NOT FOR INJECTION.

NOT TO BE DILUTED WITH WATER.

DO NOT TOUCH DROPPER TIP TO ANY SURFACE SINCE THIS MAY CONTAMINATE THE SOLUTION.

Containers

Ear drops are supplied in plastic squeeze bottles or coloured fluted glass bottles fitted with a metallic screw cap and incorporating a glass dropper tube fitted with a rubber teat.

Marketed Formulations

CIPLOX DPS (Cipla)	CANDIBIOTIC (Glenmark)
CANDID DPS (Glenmark)	GENTICYN-B (Allergan)

EXPERIMENT 80

Chloramphenicol Ear Drops BPC

Aim

To prepare and submit 10 ml of Chloramphenicol ear drops.

Formula

Sl.No	Ingredients	Official formula	Working formula
1	Chloramphenicol	10 ml	
2	Propylene Glycol (q.s)	100 ml	

Principle

Ear drops are liquid preparations instilled into the ear with a dropper. The drugs are dissolved in a suitable vehicle like water, dilute alcohol, glycerin or propylene glycol.

They are generally used for treating mild infections, softening wax and for cleansing after infections.

Chloramphenicol has poorly solubility in water and good solubility in propylene glycol. Hence to obtain a solution of effective strength, propylene glycol is used as the solvent. Chloramphenicol is used to treat mild infections of the ear.

Procedure

1. Chloramphenicol was dissolved in a small quantity of propylene glycol.
2. Propylene glycol was added to produce the required volume.

Category

Antibiotic (to treat mild infections) and Antiseptic.

Direction

Instill 1- 2 drops into the affected ear, twice or thrice a day or as advised by the physician.

Auxiliary label

FOR EXTERNAL USE ONLY.

NOT FOR INJECTION.

NOT TO BE DILUTED WITH WATER.

DO NOT TOUCH DROPPER TIP TO ANY SURFACE SINCE THIS MAY CONTAMINATE THE SOLUTION.

Storage

Store in a cool and dry place.

Marketed Formulations

CHLORAMSONE (Ranbaxy)

CLOBIOTIC (Indoco)

Nasal Drops

Nasal drops are liquid preparations for instillation into the nostrils by means of a dropper. They may be aqueous or oily solutions and usually contain medicaments with antiseptic, local analgesic and vasoconstrictor properties.

Oily drops should not be used over a long period as the oil retards the ciliary movement inside the nostrils.

Direction for Usage

1. Wipe mucus away from the nose. Older children should gently blow.
2. Tilt the head slightly back.
3. Instill 1-2 drops of the formulation into each nostril.
4. Bring the head forward and gently turn from side to side to ensure proper distribution of the solution.

Auxiliary Label

FOR EXTERNAL USE ONLY.

KEEP OUT OF REACH OF CHILDREN.

Containers

Nasal drops should be supplied in coloured fluted glass bottles fitted with a metallic screw cap and incorporating a glass dropper tube fitted with a rubber teat. Nowadays nasal drops are supplied in plastic squeeze bottles.

Marketed Formulations

OTRIVIN (Novartis)

NASIVION (Merck)

SINAREST-PD (Centaur)

EXPERIMENT 81

Ephedrine hydrochloride Nasal Drops BPC

Aim

To prepare and submit 10 ml of Ephedrine Hydrochloride Nasal drops.

Formula

Sl.No	Ingredients	Official formula	Working formula
1	Ephedrine Hydrochloride	0.5 g	
2	Chlorbutol	0.5 g	
3	Sodium Chloride	0.5 g	
4	Purified water (q.s)	100 ml	

Principle

Nasal drops are aqueous solutions meant for instillation into the nostrils by means of a dropper. They are mainly used for their antiseptic and vasoconstrictor properties. Nasal drops should be isotonic with 0.9% Sodium Chloride, pH neutral and viscosity similar to nasal secretions.

In the following preparation, the drug Ephedrine Hydrochloride is a nasal decongestant. Sodium Chloride is used to maintain isotonicity and Chlorbutol is used as a preservative. Ephedrine Hydrochloride nasal drops is used to reduce swelling of the nasal mucosa and underlying tissues in hay fever and chronic rhinitis.

Procedure

1. Ephedrine hydrochloride, sodium chloride and Chlorbutol were dissolved in a small quantity of purified water.

2. Purified water was then added to produce the required volume.

Category

To reduce swelling of the nasal mucosa and underlying tissues in hay fever and chronic rhinitis.

Method of administration

1. Wipe mucus away from the nose. Older children should gently blow.

2. Tilt the head slightly back.

3. Instill 1-2 drops of the formulation into each nostril.

4. Bring the head forward and gently turn from side to side to ensure proper distribution of the solution.

Dosage

Instill 2-3 drops, 1-3 times daily.

Auxiliary label

NOT FOR INFANTS AND CHILDREN.

FOR EXTERNAL USE ONLY.

NOT FOR INJECTION.

KEEP OUT OF REACH OF CHILDREN.

Storage

Store in a cool and dry place.

Marketed Formulations

ENDRINE (Wyeth)

ENDRINE MILD (Wyeth)

Incompatibilities

Incompatibility may be defined as the result of mixing 2 or more antagonistic substances and an undesirable product is formed which may affect the safety, efficacy and appearance of the preparation.

There are 3 types of incompatibilities:

Physical incompatibilities

Chemical incompatibilities

Therapeutic incompatibilities

Physical Incompatibilities

When 2 or more antagonistic substances are combined together, a physical change takes place and an unacceptable product is formed due to immiscibility, insolubility or liquefaction. The changes are visible and can be corrected by the application of pharmaceutical skill to obtain a product of uniform dosage, and attractive appearance.

Chemical Incompatibilities

Are caused by pH changes, complex formation, oxidation - reduction, hydrolysis or combination reactions. These reactions are noticed by precipitation, effervescence, decomposition, colour change or explosion.

Therapeutic Incompatibilities

May be a result of prescribing certain drugs to a patient with the intention to produce a specific degree of pharmacological action , but the nature or intensity of action produced is different from that intended by the prescriber.

EXPERIMENT 82

Mixtures with Physical Incompatibilities

Immiscibility

Castor oil	15 ml
Water (q.s)	100 ml

Incompatibility: Oil & water do not mix.

Remedy: Therefore carry out emulsification by the addition of an emulsifying agent.

Insolubility

Phenacetin	3.33 g
Caffeine	1.11 g
Orange syrup	13.3 ml
Water (q.s)	100 ml

Incompatibility: Phenacetin is an indiffusible solid.

Remedy: Compound powder of tragacanth (2g /100ml of finished product) or tragacanth mucilage is used as suspending agent.

It increases the viscosity of the preparation and helps to maintain uniform distribution of the insoluble substances for sufficiently long time after shaking the bottle in order to facilitate removal of a uniform dose.

Liquefaction

Menthol	130 mg
Camphor	260 mg
Light magnesium oxide	390 mg

Incompatibility: When 2 organic substances having a low melting point are brought into physical contact with each other, they liquefy due to the formation of a new substance that has a melting point below room temperature. The reason for this change is that each ingredient acts as an impurity for the other, resulting in the lowering of the melting point of both the ingredients below room temperature and the mixture liquefies. Such substances are called "Eutectic substances". E.g. Menthol & camphor.

Remedy: Eutectic powders may be dispensed in two ways:

- Dispense as separate set of powders, with directions that one set of each powder may be taken as a single dose.

- They can also be dispensed by adding an inert substance such as kaolin, starch, lactose or light magnesium oxide. These substances act as adsorbents and prevent liquefaction.

EXPERIMENT 83

Mixtures with Chemical Incompatibilities

Alkaloidal salts with alkaline substances

Alkaloids are weak bases. They are slightly soluble or insoluble in water but Alkaloidal salts are soluble in water.

If these salts are dispensed with alkaline preparations such as strong ammonia solution or ammonium bicarbonate, the free alkaloid may be precipitated out.

E.g.,	Strychnine hydrochloride solution	5 ml
	Aromatic spirit of ammonia	3.332 ml
	Water (q.s)	100 ml

Incompatibility: Strychnine hydrochloride is an Alkaloidal salt whereas Aromatic spirit of ammonia is an alkaline substance. When they both react, strychnine gets precipitated because the quantity of Strychnine hydrochloride prescribed is more than its solubility in water. This preparation contains negligible amount of alcohol which cannot dissolve strychnine. Hence it gets precipitated as diffusible precipitate.

Remedy: The following method is suitable for **diffusible** precipitates.

Divide the vehicle into 2 portions. The reactants are dissolved in separate portions and mixed slowly by adding one to the other with rapid stirring.

235

Alkaloidal salts with salicylates

E.g.,	Quinine hydrochloride	1.2 g
	Sodium salicylate	2.4 g
	Water (q.s)	100 ml

Incompatibility: When quinine compounds are combined with salicylates, indiffusible precipitates of quinine salicylate are formed.

Remedy: The following method is suitable for **indiffusible** precipitates.

Divide the vehicle into 2 portions. The first reactant is dissolved in the first portion.

Suitable amount of Compound Tragacanth powder is weighed (2g/100ml of the finished product) into a mortar and triturated with the second portion of the vehicle to form a smooth mucilage. The second reactant is dissolved in this mucilage and adjusted to suitable volume. The first mixture is then slowly added to the second mixture with rapid stirring.

Soluble salicylates with ferric salts

E.g.,	Ferric chloride solution	2 ml
	Sodium salicylate	3 g
	Water (q.s)	100 ml

Incompatibility: Ferric salts react with sodium salicylate to liberate indiffusible precipitates of ferric salicylate.

Remedy: The following method is suitable for **indiffusible** precipitates.

Divide the vehicle into 2 portions. The first reactant is dissolved in the first portion.

Suitable amount of Compound Tragacanth powder is weighed (2g/100ml of the finished product) into a mortar and triturated with the second portion of the vehicle to form a smooth mucilage. The second reactant is dissolved in this mucilage and adjusted to suitable volume. The first mixture is then slowly added to the second mixture with rapid stirring.

Or

Sodium bicarbonate is added to the preparation. In the presence of sodium bicarbonate, the precipitates of sodium salicylate remain soluble to form a clear mixture.

Soluble salicylates with alkali bicarbonates

E.g.,	Sodium salicylate	10 g
	Sodium bicarbonate	4 g
	Chloroform water (q.s)	100 ml

Incompatibility: If sodium salicylate solutions are dispensed with alkaline substances like sodium bicarbonate, the mixture undergoes oxidation (by absorbing oxygen) and turns reddish brown. This does not change the therapeutic efficacy of the mixture, but may lead to anxiety in the patient.

Remedy: A dark colouring agent like liquorice liquid extract may be added.

Or

An antioxidant such as Sodium metabisulphite (0.1%) can be added to prevent oxidation.

Soluble salicylates and benzoates with acids

Most acids and acid syrups decompose sodium salicylate or sodium benzoate to form precipitates of salicylic acid & benzoic acid respectively.

E.g.,	Sodium salicylate	5.01 g
	Lemon syrup	25 ml
	Water (q.s)	100 ml

Incompatibility: Lemon syrup contains citric acid. When it reacts with sodium salicylate, indiffusible precipitates of salicylic acid are formed.

Remedy: The following method is suitable for indiffusible precipitates.

Divide the vehicle into 2 portions. The first reactant is dissolved in the first portion.

Suitable amount of Compound Tragacanth powder is weighed (2g/100ml of the finished product) into a mortar and triturated with the second portion of the vehicle to form smooth mucilage. The second reactant is dissolved in this mucilage and adjusted to suitable volume. The first mixture is then slowly added to the second mixture with rapid stirring.

Or

Replace lemon syrup with a mixture of plain syrup and Tincture of lemon.

Incompatibility leading to evolution of CO_2

Incompatibility: When carbonates or bicarbonates & acidic drugs are dispensed in a mixture along with water, they react together leading to the evolution of CO_2.

Remedy: To prevent container leakage or explosion, the reaction must be completed before the preparation is transferred to the container. The ingredients are mixed in an open vessel & the effervescence reaction is allowed to complete after which it is transferred.

E.g.,	Sodium bicarbonate	4 g
	Borax	2 g
	Glycerol	20 ml
	Water (q.s)	100 ml

Incompatibility: When borax & glycerol are mixed together, hydrolysis of borax takes place with the formation of boric acid.

$$Na_2B_4O_7 + 3H_2O \longrightarrow Na_2B_2O_4 + 2H_3BO_3$$

Borax   sodium metaborate   boric acid

Boric acid reacts with glycerol to form monobasic glyceryl boric acid

$$2\ C_3H_5(OH)_3 + 3H_3BO_3 \longrightarrow (C_3H_5)_2(HBO_3)_3 + 6H_2O$$

Glycerol   Glyceryl boric acid

The glyceryl boric acid further reacts with sodium bicarbonate to evolve CO_2.

$$(C_3H_5)_2(HBO_3)_3 + NaHCO_3 \longrightarrow CO_2 + H_2O \uparrow$$

Glyceryl boric acid

Remedy: All the ingredients are mixed; effervescence is allowed to take place. Once it stops, it is transferred to the container.

Herapathite reaction (Quinine sulphate with iodides)

E.g.,	Quinine sulphate	5 g
	Dilute sulphuric acid	10 ml
	Potassium iodide	1.5 g
	Water (q.s)	100 ml

Incompatibility: Quinine sulphate is not freely soluble in water. It is made soluble in the presence of dilute sulphuric acid. The sulphuric acid liberates hydroiodic acid from the potassium iodide and the hydroiodic acid is partly oxidized by sulphuric acid, yielding iodine.

The iodine, hydroiodic acid and quinine sulphate then combine to form a compound called "Herapathite or iodosulphate of quinine". The mixture formed is quite clear at first, but after about 3 days, it may deposit bronze or olive green scales which are due to herapath reaction for quinine.

Herapath Reaction

$$\text{Sulphuric acid + potassium iodide} \xrightarrow{\text{Oxidation}} \text{Hydroiodic acid}$$

$$\text{Hydroiodic acid} \xrightarrow{\substack{\text{Partial oxidation by} \\ \text{Sulphuric acid}}} \text{Iodine}$$

$$\begin{array}{l}\text{Iodine + Hydroiodic acid} \\ \text{+ Quinine sulphate}\end{array} \longrightarrow \begin{array}{l}\text{Herapathite or iodosulphate of} \\ \text{Quinine which occurs as bronze or} \\ \text{olive green scales.}\end{array}$$

Remedy: To avoid any problem, only about 3 days supply should be given to the patient.

Or

The mixture should be divided, sending the potassium iodide in one bottle and Quinine sulphate in another bottle. The patient should be advised to mix both the solutions and take the necessary dose.

Soluble iodides with potassium chlorate

E.g.,	Potassium chlorate	2.22 g
	Syrup of ferric iodide	27.8 ml
	Water(q.s)	100 ml

Incompatibility: The ferric iodide is oxidized by potassium chlorate and the reaction is as follows.

$$KClO_3 + 3FeI_3 \longrightarrow 3\,FeOI + 3I_2 + KCl$$

Remedy: The mixture is clear when freshly prepared but deposit crystals of iodine upon storage for sometime. So the 2 reacting substances must be dispensed in separate bottles with a label indicating "Mix the contents of both the bottles before use".

Potassium chlorate and oxidisable substances

E.g.	Potassium chlorate	0.6 g
	Tannic acid	0.3 g
	Sucrose	0.3 g

Incompatibility: When potassium chlorate (oxidizing agent) is triturated or heated with readily oxidisable substances (reducing agents) such as charcoal, sulphur or tannic acid, there are chances of an explosion.

Remedy: Potassium chlorate and tannic acid are triturated individually. Then the powders are mixed separately with half the quantities of powdered sucrose and finally they are mixed together lightly using a spatula.

Soluble Barbiturates with Ammonium Bromide

Incompatibility: This particular combination is prescribed for the sedative action of the bromide ion of the ammonium bromide. But when ammonium bromide reacts with soluble barbiturates, it will form the poorly soluble barbitone.

This reaction can be illustrated as follows:

Phenobarbitone + Ammonium $\longrightarrow$ Phenobarbitone + Sodium
Sodium   Bromide   bromide

Remedy: Hence, to avoid this chemical reaction and without altering the therapeutic value of the prescription we have to replace ammonium bromide with equivalent amount of sodium bromide.

EXPERIMENT 84

Therapeutic Incompatibilities

Error in dosage

Rx

   Codeine Phosphate   0.5g (500 mg)

Incompatibility: The dose of Codeine is only 5 mg, but 500mg has been prescribed.

Remedy: Refer back to prescriber.

Wrong drug

 E.g.,   Drugs which have similar names

      Prednisone & Prednisolone

      Digoxin & Digitoxin

      Quinine & Quinidine

Contraindicated Drugs

E.g. penicillins and sulpha drugs are contraindicated in patients who are allergic to it.

Synergistic & antagonistic drugs

If 2 drugs which when prescribed together, increase the activity of each other. It is known as synergism.

E.g., Combination of Aspirin & Paracetamol increases analgesic activity.

Combination of Amphetamine sulphate & Ephedrine sulphate increases sympathomimetic activity.

When 2 drugs have opposing pharmacological activity, it is called antagonism.

E.g., Aspirin & Probenicid.

Drug Interactions

The effect of one drug is altered by the prior or simultaneous administration of another drug.

E.g., Tetracycline hydrochloride is inactivated by Ca^{2+} present in milk.

APPENDIX 1

Definitions of Selected Drug Categories

1. *Absorbent:* a drug that binds other chemicals into its substance, used to reduce the free availability of toxic chemicals.

2. *Abradent :* an agent that removes an external layer, such as dental plaque.

3. *Adsorbent:* a drug that binds other chemicals onto its surface, used to reduce the free availability of toxic chemicals.

4. *Alkalinizer, Systemic:* a drug that raises internal body pH, useful in restoring normal pH in patients with systemic acidosis.

5. *Analgesic:* a drug that relieves pain, without inducing unconsciousness.

6. *Antacid:* a drug that neutralizes excess gastric acid.

7. *Anesthetic, General:* a drug that eliminates pain perception by inducing unconsciousness.

8. *Anesthetic, Local:* a drug that eliminates pain perception in a limited body area by local action on sensory nerves.

9. *Anesthetic, Topical:* a local anesthetic that is effective upon application to mucous membranes.

10. *Anorexic:* a drug that suppresses appetite usually by elevating mood.

11. *Anthelmintic:* a drug that eradicates intestinal worm infestations.

12. *Antiamoebic:* a drug that kills or inhibits protozoan parasites such as *Entamoeba histolytica*, causative agent of amoebiasis.

13. *Antirachitic:* a drug with Vitamin D activity, useful for treating Vitamin D deficiency and rickets.

14. *Antibacterial:* a drug that kills or inhibits pathogenic bacteria.

15. *Anticoagulant:* a drug administered to prevent clotting.

16. *Antidiarrhoeal:* a drug that inhibits intestinal peristalsis, used to treat diarrhea.

17. *Antibiotic:* a drug, originally of microbial origin used to kill or inhibit bacterial and other infections.

18. *Antidote:* a drug that reduces the effects of a systemic poison.

19. *Antidiabetic:* a drug that supplies insulin or stimulates secretion of insulin and is useful in treating diabetes mellitus.

20. *Antidiuretic:* a drug that promotes renal water reabsorption, thus reducing urine volume, and is used to treat Diabetes insipidus.

21. *Antiemetic :* a drug that suppresses nausea and vomiting.

22. *Antienuretic:* a drug that aids in control of bedwetting (enuresis).

23. *Antiflatulent:* a drug that reduces gastrointestinal gas.

24. *Antifungal:* a drug that kills or inhibits pathogenic fungi.

25. *Antihypertensive:* a drug that lowers arterial blood pressure, especially the elevated diastolic pressure of hypertension.

26. *Antihyperlipidemic:* a drug that lowers plasma cholesterol and lipid levels.

27. *Anti- inflammatory:* a drug that inhibits or reduces inflammation.

28. *Antiperistaltic:* a drug that inhibits intestinal motility; an Antidiarrhoeal drug.

29. *Antipruritic:* a drug that reduces or relieves itching (Pruritus).

30. *Antipyretic:* a drug that restores normal body temperature in the presence of a fever (pyrexia).

31. *Antiscorbutic:* a drug with Vitamin C activity, useful in treating Vitamin C deficiency and scurvy.

32. *Antitussive:* a drug that suppresses coughing.

33. *Antiseptic:* an agent that destroys or inhibits the growth of microorganisms when applied on a wound thereby preventing infection.

34. *Astringent:* a drug used topically to toughen and shrink tissues. They cause cells to shrink by precipitating proteins from their surfaces.

35. *Anxiolytic:* a drug that suppresses symptoms of anxiety.

36. *Bronchodilator:* a drug that expands bronchiolar airways, useful in treating asthma.

37. *Carminative:* An agent that expels gases formed in the stomach or intestine.

38. *Cathartic:* a drug that promotes defecation, usually considered stronger in action than a laxative.

39. *Counter irritant:* are agents applied locally to irritate the intact skin thus reducing or relieving another irritation or deep seated pain.

40. *Demulcent:* a bland viscous liquid, usually water based, used to coat and soothe damaged or inflamed skin or mucous membranes.

41. *Diagnostic aid:* a drug used to determine the functional state of a body organ or to determine the presence of a disease.

42. *Diaphoretic:* a drug that increases sweating to bring down elevated body temperatures.

43. *Digestive aid:* a drug that promotes digestion, usually by supplementing a gastrointestinal enzyme.

44. *Disinfectant:* an agent that destroys microorganisms on contact and suitable for sterilizing inanimate objects.

45. *Diuretic:* a drug that promotes renal excretion of electrolytes and water, useful in treating generalized oedema.

46. *Emetic:* a drug that induces vomiting, useful in expelling ingested but unabsorbed poisons.

47. *Emollient:* a topical drug, especially an oil or fat used to soften the skin and make it more pliable.

48. *Expectorant:* a drug that increases respiratory tract secretions lowers their viscosity and promotes removal.

49. *Hematopoietic:* a vitamin that stimulates formation of blood cells and is useful in treating vitamin deficiency anaemia.

50. *Haematinic:* a drug that promotes hemoglobin formation by supplying iron.

51. *Haemostatic:* a drug applied to a bleeding surface to promote clotting.

52. *Humectant:* is a substance that promotes retention of moisture.

53. *Hypnotic:* a central nervous system depressant used to induce sleep.

54. *Keratolytic:* a topical drug that softens the superficial keratin containing layer of the skin and promotes desquamation.

55. *Laxative:* a drug that softens hard stools and facilitates its removal from the bowel. Usually considered milder in action than a cathartic.

56. *Mucolytic:* a drug that hydrolyzes mucoproteins, useful in reducing the viscosity of pulmonary mucous.

57. *Non steroidal anti inflammatory drug (NSAID):* an analgesic, anti inflammatory drug that inhibits prostaglandin synthesis.

58. *Nasal decongestant:* an adrenergic drug used orally or topically to induce vasoconstriction in the nasal passages.

59. *Protectant:* a topical drug that provides physical barrier to the environment.

60. *Purgative:* an agent that promotes bowel evacuation with fluid stools. It is stronger than a laxative.

61. *Rubefacient:* a topical drug that induces mild skin irritation with redness and is used as a toughening agent. (They are also defined as substances that produce congestion & redness of the area to which they are applied producing the initial symptoms of irritation).

62. *Saline Purgative:* an agent that does not undergo absorption in GIT and increases the volume of the gut contents by retaining water and also by drawing fluid from the tissues, thereby stimulates peristalsis and hastens faecal evacuation.

63. *Sedative:* a CNS depressant used to induce mild relaxation. It subdues excitement and calms a person without inducing sleep.

64. *Thrombolytic:* an enzyme drug administered parenterally to solubilize blood clots.

65. *Vasodilator:* a drug that expands blood vessels.

66. *Vasoconstrictor:* a drug that narrows arterioles, usually to elevate BP.

APPENDIX 2

Preparation of Pharmaceutical Ingredients

Anise water, Concentrated: is prepared using the following formula.

Anise oil	-	20 ml
Alcohol (90%)	-	700 ml
Purified water (q.s)	-	1000 ml

Dissolve the anise oil in the alcohol and add sufficient water in small portions to produce 1000ml, shaking vigorously after each addition. Add 50g of sterilized Purified Talc or other suitable filtering aid. Shake occasionally and filter.

Amaranth Solution: is prepared using the following formula.

Amaranth	-	10 g
Chloroform water (q.s)	-	1000 ml

Benzaldehyde spirit: is prepared using the following formula.

Alcohol (90%)	-	800 ml
Benzaldehyde	-	10 ml
Purified water (q.s)	-	1000 ml

Dissolve the Benzaldehyde in the alcohol and add sufficient water to produce the required volume.

Camphor water BP: is prepared using the following formula.

Camphor	-	1 g
Alcohol (90%)	-	2 ml
Purified Water (q.s)	-	1000 ml

Dissolve the camphor in the alcohol and add sufficient water in small quantities to produce the required volume, shaking vigorously after each addition.

Camphor water, Concentrated: is prepared using the following formula.

Camphor	-	40 g
Alcohol (90%)	-	600 ml
Water (q.s)	-	1000 ml

Dissolve the camphor in the alcohol and add sufficient water in small quantities to produce the required volume, shaking vigorously after each addition.

Chloroform spirit BP: is prepared using the following formula.

Chloroform	-	50 ml
Alcohol 90% (q.s)	-	1000 ml

Mix both the ingredients.

Chloroform water BP: is prepared using the following formula.

Chloroform	-	2.5 ml
Purified water (q.s)	-	1000 ml

Dissolve the chloroform in the purified water by shaking.

Chloroform water, Double strength, BPC: is prepared using the following formula.

Chloroform	-	5 ml
Purified water (q.s)	-	1000 ml

Cinnamon   water,   Concentrated: